Alternative Healing

Series Editor: Cara Acred

Volume 269

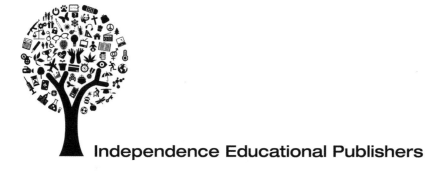

Independence Educational Publishers

First published by Independence Educational Publishers

The Studio, High Green

Great Shelford

Cambridge CB22 5EG

England

© Independence 2014

British Library Cataloguing in Publication Data

Alternative healing. -- (Issues ; 269)

1. Alternative medicine. 2. Alternative medicine--Great

Britain.

I. Series II. Acred, Cara editor.

615.5-dc23

ISBN-13: 9781861686886

Printed in Great Britain

MWL Print Group Ltd

Contents

Introduction

Alternative Healing is Volume 269 in the **ISSUES** series. The aim of the series is to offer current, diverse information about important issues in our world, from a UK perspective.

ABOUT ALTERNATIVE HEALING

Increasing numbers of people are turning to alternative and complementary medicines for help with ailments, from minor conditions to life-threatening illnesses. While many are strong proponents of the benefits of alternative healing, others remain sceptical and cite the 'placebo' effect when explaining their successes. This book explores the various techniques and therapies covered by complementary and alternative medicines (CAM), looks at how to find a reliable CAM practitioner and considers the issues and debates surrounding the use of alternative treatments.

OUR SOURCES

Titles in the **ISSUES** series are designed to function as educational resource books, providing a balanced overview of a specific subject.

The information in our books is comprised of facts, articles and opinions from many different sources, including:

⇨ Newspaper reports and opinion pieces

⇨ Website factsheets

⇨ Magazine and journal articles

⇨ Statistics and surveys

⇨ Government reports

⇨ Literature from special interest groups.

A NOTE ON CRITICAL EVALUATION

Because the information reprinted here is from a number of different sources, readers should bear in mind the origin of the text and whether the source is likely to have a particular bias when presenting information (or when conducting their research). It is hoped that, as you read about the many aspects of the issues explored in this book, you will critically evaluate the information presented.

It is important that you decide whether you are being presented with facts or opinions. Does the writer give a biased or unbiased report? If an opinion is being expressed, do you agree with the writer? Is there potential bias to the 'facts' or statistics behind an article?

ASSIGNMENTS

In the back of this book, you will find a selection of assignments designed to help you engage with the articles you have been reading and to explore your own opinions. Some tasks will take longer than others and there is a mixture of design, writing and research-based activities that you can complete alone or in a group.

FURTHER RESEARCH

At the end of each article we have listed its source and a website that you can visit if you would like to conduct your own research. Please remember to critically evaluate any sources that you consult and consider whether the information you are viewing is accurate and unbiased.

Useful weblinks

www.acupuncture.org.uk

www.alzheimers.org.uk

www.anh-europe.org

www.cambrella.eu

www.cancerresearchuk.org

www.theconversation.com

www.drjessamy.com

www.nhs.uk

www.patient.co.uk

www.therapy-directory.org.uk

www.traffic.org

www.whatmedicine.co.uk

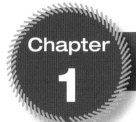

Chapter 1

Complementary medicine

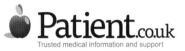

Patient.co.uk
Trusted medical information and support

Complementary and alternative medicine

Complementary and alternative medicine (CAM) includes a group of diverse medical and healthcare systems, practices, and products that are not generally considered part of conventional medicine. Complementary medicine is generally regarded as a complementary treatment that is used alongside conventional medicine, whereas alternative medicine is regarded as a treatment used in place of conventional medicine.[1]

There has been considerable interest in CAM, with a House of Lords Select Committee Report in November 2000 and a subcommittee of the Royal College of Physicians set up to examine certain aspects.[2] They reported in *Clinical Medicine* in 2003.[3]

The House of Lords Select Committee was very keen that there should be professional standards, registration and accountability in all aspects of CAM.[2] Statutory regulation of the acupuncture profession has failed to happen and it is now thought any regulation in the future will be voluntary.[4] Osteopathy is regulated by the General Osteopathic Council. Chiropractic is regulated by the General Chiropractic Council.

CAM does appeal to patients; many feel it is more natural; some feel the holistic approach benefits them; others may turn to it when they feel conventional medicine has let them down. We have a duty to help our patients make informed decisions about their healthcare. We should provide them with the evidence about CAM to aid their empowerment and decision-making process. High-quality evidence is often lacking and a UK study (looking at the impact of CAM on health outcomes) called for those evaluating impact, to use standardised tools to improve the overall quality of the studies.[5]

Complementary and alternative medicine use

A report in the *Lancet* in 2007 stated that about 13,000 patients had been treated at four homeopathic hospitals (Bristol, Glasgow, Liverpool and London) in the UK each year.[6] 14.5% of the population say that they trust homeopathy and £38 million is spent on homeopathy each year in the UK.

Of the various forms of CAM, acupuncture is amongst the most popular. Approximately three million people undergo acupuncture treatment in the UK each year.[7]

Homeopathy

Homeopathic treatment is still available within the NHS; however, not all primary care trusts or GPs agree to fund referrals.[8]

The homeopathic approach is based on the concept that 'like cures like' – in other words, that 'an illness can be treated with a substance, taken in small amounts, that produces similar symptoms in a healthy person'.[9] For example, the homeopathic remedy allium cepa is made from an extract of onions. If a person chops onions, they make the eyes sting and water and the nose run. Using the homeopathic philosophy of 'like for like', this means that a disorder with these symptoms should be cured by a small dose of onion. Hence, allium cepa may be used to treat hay fever.

Homeopathic medicines are prepared by serial dilution in steps of 1:10 or 1:100, denoted by the Latin numbers x and c, respectively. At each step there is succussion, or vigorous shaking. The dilution most frequently sold in pharmacies is 6c, which is a 10–12 dilution of the original mother tincture. Hence, it is likely that a 6c dilution will contain just a few molecules of the initial substance, but much higher dilutions, such as the 30c (10–60), will contain even fewer.

One of the leading proposals for how such 'ultramolecular' dilutions work is the 'information hypothesis'. This is the theory that water is capable of storing information relating to substances with which it has previously been in contact, and subsequently transmitting this information to biosystems.[10] There is some research from the field of materials science suggesting that this is plausible.[11] Succussion has been suggested as an important part of this process.

There have been many publications and much debate and controversy about the evidence for homeopathy. On the whole, meta-analyses of homeopathy are inconclusive and don't provide

1 What Is Complementary and Alternative Medicine? National Center for Complementary and Alternative Medicine, last updated July 2011.

2 House of Lords Select Committee on Science and Technology. 6th report, session 1999-2000. Complementary and alternative medicine. November 2000.

3 Lewith GT, Breen A, Filshie J, et al; Complementary medicine: evidence base, competence to practice and regulation. Clin Med. 2003 May-Jun;3(3):235-40.

4 British Acupuncture Council; BAcC represents acupuncturists trained in traditional acupuncture in the United Kingdom.

5 Wye L, Sharp D, Shaw A; The impact of NHS based primary care complementary therapy services on health BMC Complement Altern Med. 2009 Mar 6;9:5.

6 Samarasekera U; Pressure grows against homeopathy in the UK. Lancet. 2007 Nov 17;370(9600):1677-8.

7 Effective Health Care. Acupuncture. An objective assessment (from the York Centre and published by the Royal Society of Medicine). Centre for reviews and dissemination, University of York; Vol. 7 No. 2, Nov 2001.

8 Kmietowicz Z; NHS should stop funding homoeopathy, MPs say. BMJ 2010; 340:c1091.

9 British Homeopathic Association and Faculty of Homeopathy.

10 Lewith GT et al; Complementary medicine: evidence base, competence to practice and regulation. Clinical Medicine, Journal of the Royal College of Physicians, Volume 3, Number 3, 1 May 2003 , pp. 235-240(6).

11 Rao ML, Roy R, Bell IR, et al; The defining role of structure (including epitaxy) in the plausibility of Homeopathy. 2007 Jul;96(3):175-82.

sufficient information for conclusions to be drawn about homeopathy in general. Certain randomised controlled trials and clinical outcome studies have, however, shown some benefit.[12,13] It has also been suggested that the benefits of homeopathy are due to the quality and holistic nature of the homeopathic consultation, rather than to the remedies themselves.[14] Cochrane reviews (various dates and conditions) state homeopathy provides no benefit above that of placebo.

The Faculty of Homeopathy regulates the training and practise of homeopathy by medically qualified doctors. There is a published list of doctors who are members of the faculty:[15,16]

⇨ The most experienced homeopaths have the qualifications FFHom or MFHom.

⇨ The qualification LFHom indicates a doctor who may use homeopathy in a limited way for minor ailments.

For homeopaths who are not doctors, there is no single registering body. The Society of Homeopaths is the largest professional organisation registering homeopaths in Britain. It has more than 2,300 members who must satisfy the Society's code of practice.

Acupuncture

Acupuncture originated in China, probably more than 4,000 years ago. The profession has robust self-regulation by the British Acupuncture Council and this has been acknowledged by Parliament.[4] The house of Lords Select Committee on Science and Technology defined acupuncture as follows:[17]

'Acupuncture involves inserting small needles into various points in the body to stimulate nerve impulses. Traditional Chinese acupuncture is based on the idea of "qi" (vital energy) which is said to travel around the body along

12 Shang A, Huwiler-Muntener K, Nartey L, et al; Are the clinical effects of homoeopathy placebo effects? Comparative study of placebo-controlled trials of homoeopathy and allopathy.; Lancet. 2005 Aug 27-Sep 2;366(9487):726-32.

13 Nuhn T, Ludtke R, Geraedts M; Placebo effect sizes in homeopathic compared to conventional drugs - a systematic Homeopathy. 2010 Jan;99(1):76-82.

14 Hartog CS; Elements of effective communication--rediscoveries from homeopathy. Patient Educ Couns. 2009 Nov;77(2):172-8. Epub 2009 Apr 15.

15 Introduction to Homeopathy, NHS Evidence - CAM; NHS library information on complementary and alternative medicine.

16 Complementary medicine: information for primary care clinicians, Dept of Health, June 2000.

17 Sixth Report. Complementary and Alternative Medicine, House of Lords Select Committee on Science and Technology, November 2000.

"meridians" which the acupuncture points affect. Western acupuncture uses the same needling technique but is based on affecting nerve impulses and the central nervous system; acupuncture may be used in the West as an anaesthetic agent and also as an analgesic.'

Numerous Cochrane reviews have looked at the evidence for acupuncture in certain conditions. Many reviews conclude that further analysis is required, but the following have more positive conclusions:

⇨ Headache: acupuncture could be a valuable non-pharmacological tool in patients with frequent episodic or chronic tension-type headaches.[18]

⇨ Migraine prophylaxis: acupuncture is at least as effective as, or possibly more effective than, prophylactic drug treatment, and has fewer adverse effects. Acupuncture should be considered a treatment option for patients willing to undergo this treatment.[19]

⇨ In vitro fertilisation (IVF) treatment: acupuncture does increase the live birth rate with IVF treatment when performed around the time of embryo transfer. Larger trials are needed.[20]

⇨ Neck pain: there is moderate evidence that acupuncture for chronic neck pain is more effective than placebo at the end of treatment and at short-term follow-up.[21]

⇨ Nausea and vomiting during chemotherapy: electro-acupuncture seems to be beneficial in treating acute vomiting induced by chemotherapy. However, it needs to be compared with the newer anti-emetics and its use in those with refractory symptoms needs investigating.[22]

⇨ Back pain: no firm conclusions can be drawn about the effectiveness

18 Linde K, Allais G, Brinkhaus B, et al; Acupuncture for tension-type headache. Cochrane Database Syst Rev. 2009 Jan 21;(1):CD007587.

19 Linde K, Allais G, Brinkhaus B, et al; Acupuncture for migraine prophylaxis. Cochrane Database Syst Rev. 2009 Jan 21;(1):CD001218.

20 Cheong YC, Hung Yu Ng E, Ledger WL; Acupuncture and assisted conception. Cochrane Database Syst Rev. 2008 Oct 8;(4):CD006920.

21 Trinh K, Graham N, Gross A, et al; Acupuncture for neck disorders.; Cochrane Database Syst Rev. 2006 Jul 19;3:CD004870.

22 Ezzo JM, Richardson MA, Vickers A, et al; Acupuncture-point stimulation for chemotherapy-induced nausea or vomiting.; Cochrane Database Syst Rev. 2006 Apr 19;(2):CD002285.

of acupuncture for acute pain but it does achieve pain relief and functional improvement in chronic low back pain and is recommended by the National Institute for Health and Clinical Excellence (NICE).[23]

⇨ Postoperative nausea and vomiting: compared with anti-emetic prophylaxis, P6 acupoint stimulation seems to reduce the risk of nausea but not vomiting postoperatively.[24]

A large prospective UK trial of 34,000 consultations found no reports of serious adverse events (defined as events requiring hospital admission, leading to permanent disability, or resulting in death).[25] Practitioners did report 43 minor adverse events. The most common events were severe nausea and fainting. There were three avoidable events; two patients had needles left in and one patient had moxibustion burns to the skin, caused by practitioners' errors.

Reflexology

The House of Lords' Select Committee on Complementary and Alternative Medicine described reflexology as follows:[17] 'A system of massage of the feet based on the idea that there are invisible zones running vertically through the body, so that each organ has a corresponding location in the foot. It has also been claimed to stimulate blood supply and relieve tension.'

The concept behind reflexology is that reflex points on the feet and hands correspond to all of the organs, glands and parts of the body. For example, the toes represent the head and the ball of the foot represents the chest and lung region.[26] By applying pressure to these points, it is thought that blood circulation is improved, the body relaxes and organs and glands become balanced.[26] There is less research on the proposed mechanism of action of reflexology than on acupuncture or manipulation. It is thought that the areas activated by massage of the feet may have something in common with the lines of 'qi' in acupuncture.

23 Low back pain; NICE Clinical guideline (May 2009).

24 Lee A, Fan LT; Stimulation of the wrist acupuncture point P6 for preventing postoperative nausea and vomiting; Cochrane Database Syst Rev. 2009 Apr 15;(2):CD003281.

25 MacPherson H, Thomas K, Walters S, et al; The York acupuncture safety study: prospective survey of 34,000 treatments by BMJ. 2001 Sep 1;323(7311):486-7.

26 International Institute of Reflexology; Website with information about reflexology and reflexology training.

The Database of Abstracts of Reviews of Effects (DARE) discussed a review in 2001 that looked at the existing literature on reflexology.[27] Seven trials were included in the review, five of which were randomised. However, there were only 214 participants in total and the authors of the review concluded that, of those trials that had been published on reflexology, 'all are methodologically flawed and their results are non-uniform. The effectiveness of reflexology is not supported by controlled clinical trials.' They suggested that more research was needed to establish specific effects.

Manipulation therapies – osteopathy and chiropractic

The 'manipulative therapies' include osteopathy and chiropractic. The two therapies have some similarities. Their practitioners use their hands to work with joints, muscles and connective tissue and to diagnose and treat soft tissue imbalances and abnormalities in skeletal function. Manipulation techniques are commonly used for low back pain, neck pain, shoulder pain, headache and sports injuries.

Osteopathy is regulated by the General Osteopathic Council. Chiropractic is regulated by the General Chiropractic Council. The practices were first introduced into the UK in the late 19th century.[28,29]

Some common techniques used by both osteopaths and chiropractors include:[28]

⇨ High-velocity thrusts: a short, sharp controlled movement with low amplitude is applied to the spine to restore local articular range and quality of movement. This produces the classic 'cracking' sound.

⇨ Muscle energy technique: a soft tissue technique to increase a joint's range of movement.

⇨ Functional technique: taking a joint into continuous, different planes of movement that produce little tension and do not provoke pain. The idea is eventually to work back to the initial starting position – now, it is hoped, with less or no pain. This technique reduces the stimulation through the local

neuromuscular tissues and can lead to a release in tension.

Much has been made of the potential dangers of spinal manipulation but (despite its widespread use) serious complications seldom occur. The risk of a serious complication due to manipulation is somewhere between one in 100,000[30] and one in 5.8 million.[29,31]

Where there have been problems from manipulation, they have more often been when manipulating the cervical spine.[29]

The following are contra-indications to manipulation at any level:

⇨ Any potential sinister cause of back pain, including a history of malignancy that may involve bone, such as breast cancer or a haematological malignancy.

⇨ A patient on anticoagulants or who has a clotting disorder.[32] Some suggest that this is a relative contra-indication and depends on the patient's age and where the practitioner is wanting to manipulate. Cervical spine manipulation carries a higher risk. Thoracic and lumbar spine manipulation carries a lower risk, especially in a younger patient.

⇨ A patient with neurological disease. Manipulation is contra-indicated if there are upper motor neurone signs. However, some practitioners would be happy to perform manipulation at adjacent joints in those with lower motor neurone signs, in order to unload the strain at the nerve root affected.

⇨ Presence of cauda equina syndrome.

⇨ Active inflammatory arthritis.

The evidence for manipulation for back pain:

⇨ The UK 'back pain, exercise and manipulation' (BEAM) trial was a randomised trial based on 181

general practices.[33] It concluded that spinal manipulation is a cost-effective addition to 'best care' for back pain in general practice. Manipulation alone probably gives better value for money than manipulation followed by exercise.

⇨ A Cochrane review in 2004 concluded that there was no evidence that spinal manipulative therapy was superior to other standard treatments for patients with acute or chronic low back pain.[34]

⇨ The European Back Pain Guidelines have recommended the use of manipulation for acute nonspecific low back pain[35] and chronic nonspecific low back pain.[36]

Aromatherapy

Aromatherapy is a complementary therapy that uses plant extract essential oils that are either inhaled, used as a massage oil, or occasionally ingested. It can be used to alleviate specific symptoms or as a relaxant.[17] It is based on the healing properties of essential oils, of which there are over 400, extracted from plants all over the world. Popular oils used include chamomile, lavender, rosemary and tea tree.[37] Aromatherapy carrier oils are used for mixing blends of essential oils in order to make bath oils or massage oils. They are mainly extracted from nuts and seeds. Examples are sweet almond oil, evening primrose oil and black seed oil.

Aromatherapy can help to promote relaxation.[38] It is currently widely used in the management of chronic pain, depression, anxiety and stress, insomnia and some cognitive disorders.[39]

Side-effects can include allergic

27 Ernst E, Koder K, An overview of reflexology, DARE – (Database of Abstracts of Reviews of Effects), Centre for reviews and dissemination, University of York.

28 Vickers A, Zollman C; ABC of complementary medicine. The manipulative therapies: osteopathy and chiropractic. BMJ. 1999 Oct 30;319(7218):1176-9.

29 Introduction to Osteopathy, NHS National Library for Health, last updated Dec 2009.

30 Rothwell DM, Bondy SJ, Williams JI; Chiropractic manipulation and stroke: a population-based case-control study. Stroke. 2001 May;32(5):1054-60.

31 Haldeman S, Carey P, Townsend M, et al; Arterial dissections following cervical manipulation: the chiropractic experience. CMAJ. 2001 Oct 2;165(7):905-6.

32 Whedon JM, Quebada PB, Roberts DW, et al; Spinal epidural hematoma after spinal manipulative therapy in a patient undergoing anticoagulant therapy: a case report. J Manipulative Physiol Ther. 2006 Sep;29(7):582-5.

33 No authors listed; United Kingdom back pain exercise and manipulation (UK BEAM) randomised trial: cost effectiveness of physical treatments for back pain in primary care. BMJ. 2004 Dec 11;329(7479):1381. Epub 2004 Nov 19.

34 Assendelft WJ, Morton SC, Yu EI, et al; Spinal manipulative therapy for low back pain; Cochrane Database Syst Rev. 2004;(1):CD000447.

35 European guidelines for the management of acute nonspecific low back pain in primary care; COST B13 Working Group (2004).

36 European guidelines for the management of chronic non-specific low back pain, COST B13 Working Group (2004).

37 Aromatherapy Council.

38 Complementary medicine: information pack for primary care groups, Dept of Health, June 2000.

39 Perry N, Perry E; Aromatherapy in the management of psychiatric disorders: clinical and neuropharmacological perspectives. CNS Drugs. 2006;20(4):257-80.

reactions (including rash for patient or therapist[40]), headache and nausea. It should also be noted that:[41]

⇨ Patients with diabetes should avoid angelica.

⇨ Patients with epilepsy should avoid fennel, rosemary and sage (because of the risk of over-stimulating the nervous system).

⇨ Patients with hypertension should avoid hyssop, rosemary, sage and thyme.

⇨ Pregnant ladies should avoid basil, laurel, angelica, thyme, cumin, aniseed, citronella and juniper. An aromatherapist should always be alerted if the patient is pregnant because of potential teratogenic and uterine effects of the oils.

⇨ Those with sensitive skins should avoid basil, laurel, coriander, tea tree, neroli, geranium, mint, yarrow, Roman and German chamomile, lemon balm, citronella, ginger, hops, jasmine, lemon, lemon grass (unless greatly diluted with a carrier oil), turmeric and valerian. Skin patch testing can be carried out beforehand if there are concerns. Care should be taken in those with a history of allergy or atopic conditions such as asthma, eczema or hayfever.

⇨ Oestrogen-dependent tumours such as breast cancer or ovarian cancer, are a contra-indication to the use of oils with oestrogen-like compounds, such as fennel, aniseed, sage, and clary sage.

⇨ There may be possible interactions of essential oils, with antibiotics, antihistamines and sedatives.

⇨ Cinnamon, turmeric, valerian, laurel, juniper, aniseed, coriander and eucalyptus should not be used for longer than two weeks at a time because of concerns about toxicity.

⇨ Bitter almond, red thyme, common sage, rue, wormwood, tansy, savory, wintergreen and sassafras oils should be avoided at all times by everyone as they can be poisonous.

A review in the *British Journal of General Practice* in 2000 found

12 trials of aromatherapy.[42] It concluded that:

⇨ The studies suggested that aromatherapy massage has a mild, transient anxiolytic effect.

⇨ The effects of aromatherapy are probably not strong enough for it to be considered for the treatment of anxiety.

⇨ The hypothesis that it is effective for any other indication is not supported by the findings of rigorous clinical trials.

Herbal remedies

The medicinal properties of herbs have been exploited for many centuries. The druids and the Ancient Egyptians are amongst the best known exponents of herbal medicine. The concern is that many herbal remedies that are for sale have not been thoroughly tested for efficacy, toxicity, drug interactions and teratogenicity. In addition, there are often problems of variation in potency between batches and correct doses are not carefully established.

The Medicines and Healthcare products Regulatory Agency (MHRA) is the government agency which is responsible for ensuring that medicines and medical devices work, and are acceptably safe.[43] The MHRA website also provides a list of herbal ingredients which are prohibited or restricted in medicines.

Hypnosis

Hypnosis may be practised by medically qualified people, clinical psychologists or those without healthcare qualifications. Hypnosis must be used with skill and care, as adverse events, including the implantation of false memories, may occur. The British Society of Clinical Hypnosis can help in finding a registered practitioner.[44] Both competence and ethics are essential.

Examples of conditions amenable to treatment include:

⇨ Smoking cessation.

⇨ Weight control.

⇨ Irrational fears and phobias.

⇨ Stress management.

⇨ Compulsive behaviour.

42 Cooke B, Ernst E; Aromatherapy: a systematic review. Br J Gen Pract. 2000 Jun;50(455):493-6.

43 Using herbal medicines safely, Medicines and Healthcare products Regulatory Agency, accessed March 2012.

44 British Society of Clinical Hypnosis; their aim is to promote and assure high standards in the hypnotherapy profession.

⇨ Anxiety and panic attacks.

There have been a number of systematic reviews, including Cochrane reviews of the various topics.

Macrobiotic diets

The aim of the macrobiotic diet is to avoid foods containing toxins. It is a completely vegan diet and no dairy products or meats are allowed. Macrobiotic diets have become popular with people who have cancer who believe that it can help them fight their cancer and lead to a cure. However, as yet there is no scientific evidence supporting a macrobiotic diet treating or curing cancer or any other disease.[45]

Chelation therapy

Chelation therapy is the use of chelating agents – usually the man-made amino acid ethylene diamine tetra-acetic acid (EDTA) – to remove heavy metals from the body. It is of proven value in Wilson's disease, haemochromatosis and heavy metal poisoning (including lead and mercury). However, it has also been promoted by some for the treatment of other disorders, including arterial disease, Alzheimer's disease and autism.

Faith healing

Faith healing is not new. It is well documented in both the Old Testament (Second Book of Kings, chapter 5) and New Testament (Gospel of Luke, chapter 8, verses 26 to 56) of the Bible, along with the observation that it is only effective where there is absolute faith. There are still charismatic preachers who carry out 'faith' healing in which people come to the front and publicly discard the wheelchairs that they have allegedly depended upon for many years.

Conclusion

There is some evidence that CAM may work for certain conditions but, for many conditions, the evidence is of poor quality and it is impossible to draw a firm conclusion about its effectiveness. However, we must remember that this is not the same as evidence of lack of efficacy. More research is needed in this area.

⇨ Used with permission from Patient.co.uk, available at http://www.patient.co.uk/doctor/complementary-and-alternative-medicine.

40 Trattner A, David M, Lazarov A; Occupational contact dermatitis due to essential oils. Contact Dermatitis. 2008 May;58(5):282-4.

41 Safe Alternative Medicine; Expert advice on alternative medicine, accessed March 2012.

45 Macrobiotic diet, CancerHelp UK.

Evolving use of alternative medicines

Alternative medicines will continue to influence healthcare decisions in many societies out to 2050. Alternative medicine is growing in popularity: homeopathic medicine, for example, is a more than one billion/year industry. Meanwhile, Western medicine faces up to ominous consequences for decades of antibiotic and pain medication overuse. A preferable future outcome may represent an integrated version of both Western and alternative care that avoids extreme positions on good health.

In Canada for example, alternative, or complementary, medicine used for chronic conditions in pediatrics is on the rise. Chronic illnesses in children like asthma and obesity, globally on the rise, represent a growing market for this type of treatment. Because of the expected long-term impact of these diseases on society, identifying a safe and noninvasive treatment would have huge benefits since the obesity generation is growing up into adults with expensive and debilitating health problems.

Another demographic force of change is the large Baby Boomer cohort approaching old age in an era with many alternatives to traditional medicine. Boomer open-mindedness may again prove its capacity to transform society, this time by raising the status of alternative medicine. An important artifact of the baby boomer zeitgeist is the recognition of the mind-body connection, which focused on opening the mind in their youth but perhaps may become channelled into living longer, healthier lives in their old age. An example is the Stanford study toward creating a 'virtual compassion gym' where individuals can be trained in altruism and empathy, traits which have been shown to reduce inflammation and improve cardiac function, among other benefits. Similarly, new research supports psychosomatic treatment, such as meditation, for chronic pain. Perhaps future alternative treatments will have social as well as individual health benefits, including a less drug-dependent and mindful society.

Embracing the mind-body connection also might signal the rising impact of the East on consumer culture, which will in turn grow to influence the direction of the healthcare market. As the influence of Asian consumers rises, cultural preferences will start to shape the products and services offered.

China's new middle class has more discretionary income to spend, and some of it will go to healthcare. Will Chinese healthcare consumers replace their traditional treatments with Western ones, or help advance alternatives? Meanwhile, there is an aspect of globalisation which de-stigmatises traditional remedies from non-Western/Anglo cultures. Cross-cultural exchange through globalising forces has helped advanced acceptance of differences, although it also creates many opportunities for co-opting sensitive and valued traditions. Moving toward 2050, traditional healing may gain greater acceptance and earn many more customers, but it may likely be a different interpretation.

Fragmented social organisation is another cultural force favouring the rise of alternative medicines. Disillusionment with large, private institutions, BigPharma, and other symbols of centralised knowledge and power is growing. Access to information is being broken down by the World Wide Web, so by 2050 expect to see health and healing as much more participatory and far less top-down. Information comes at a cost, though: 'cyberchondriacs' feel sicker with each Google search result. Reducing the anxiety that ambiguous online information creates in patients may be a part of some future medical practices or health services.

The cost of health care is expected to rise, and, some have predicted, so will economic inequality. The fact that alternative medicine is cheaper will allow it to flourish among expensive high-tech treatments. However, substituting inadequate alternative treatments or untrained practitioners for standard health care is a dangerous prospect. Regulation of alternative medicine will need to make progress by 2050: it will be likely that alternative health practitioners will supplement the shrinking workforce of medical doctors, filling the coming shortage in healthcare providers.

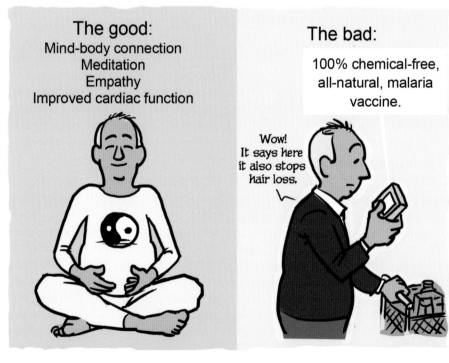

The good:
Mind-body connection
Meditation
Empathy
Improved cardiac function

The bad:
100% chemical-free, all-natural, malaria vaccine.

Wow! It says here it also stops hair loss.

Meanwhile, there are major red flags about the 'end of antibiotics' that suggest shying away from pharmaceutical treatments could be wise. Studies by the Centers for Disease Control found that antibiotic-resistant outbreaks quadrupled in the span of a decade in the U.S. Public health experts in the UK and in the WHO have also spoken out about the increasingly emergent crisis in bacterial infections, called 'apocalyptic' and a 'nightmare'. Without the discovery of new antibiotics or some other strategy to outsmart the resistant bacteria, this is an unavoidable image of the global future that is for now very bleak. The rise of the antibiotic-resistant infection is a major uncertainty in health going forward to 2050.

What does it all mean for the future of alternative medicines?

The technological advances with promise for the future of healthcare, such as stem cell therapy and robotics, while innovative, will usher in an era of medical care that is extremely high-tech. Meanwhile, the superbug ticking time bomb could blow up and end the era of medical miracles through antibiotics. Backlash toward medical science could steer consumers toward alternative treatment: herbs, body work, pressure points and homeopathics among others. In fact, if antibiotics are ineffective, there may be few other choices than folk remedies. The superbug crisis could awaken a reverence for lost and ancient human wisdom, which alternative medicines might symbolise.

The future of alternative healthcare deals with tensions between wisdom and knowledge; it seems to put tradition and technology at odds. Instead, why not imagine that 2050 would offer solutions to extreme viewpoints that discount one school (science or tradition) in favour of the other. Perhaps more caution could have prevented our arrival at the antibiotic apocalypse. Balance is much more desirable in the future of healthcare, so by 2050 there may be a good number of options to choose from both high-tech and alternative treatments if good decisions can be implemented soon.

⇨ The above information is reprinted with kind permission from the European Commission. Please visit ec.europa.eu for further information.

© European Commission 2014

The difference between complementary and alternative therapies

This article has information about complementary therapies used by people with cancer and the difference between complementary and alternative therapies.

The difference between complementary and alternative therapies

The phrases complementary therapy and alternative therapy are often used as if they mean the same thing. They may also be combined into one phrase – complementary and alternative therapies, or CAMs. It is not always easy to decide whether something is a complementary or an alternative therapy. But there is an important difference.

A complementary therapy means you can use it alongside your conventional medical treatment. It may help you to feel better and cope better with your cancer and treatment. It is important to discuss with your doctor any complementary therapy that you are thinking of using.

An alternative therapy is generally used instead of conventional medical treatment. All conventional cancer treatments have to go through rigorous testing by law in order to prove that they work. Most alternative therapies have not been through such testing and there is no scientific evidence that they work. Some types of alternative therapy may not be completely safe and could cause harmful side-effects.

If you are thinking of using CAMs

If you are considering using any complementary or alternative therapy it is very important to talk to your cancer doctor, GP, or specialist nurse for advice about the safety of the therapy. It is also very important to let your complementary or alternative therapist know about your conventional cancer treatment.

What complementary therapies are

Complementary therapies are used alongside conventional medical treatments prescribed by your doctor. They can help people with cancer to feel better and may improve your quality of life. They may also help you to cope better with symptoms caused by the cancer or side-effects caused by cancer treatment. The following page has information about some of the reasons why people with cancer use complementary therapies.

A good complementary therapist won't claim that the therapy will cure your cancer. They would always encourage you to discuss any therapies with your cancer doctor or GP. Complementary therapies are available from many different types of people and organisations. Further on you can find out where you can have complementary therapies.

There are many different types of complementary therapy, including the following:

⇨ Aromatherapy

⇨ Acupuncture

⇨ Herbal medicine

⇨ Massage therapy

⇨ Visualisation

⇨ Yoga.

Many health professionals are very supportive of people with cancer using complementary therapies. They can see that the therapies help people to cope better with the cancer and its treatment. But some health professionals have been reluctant for their patients to use such therapies. This is because many therapies have not been scientifically tested in the same way as conventional treatments.

Some research trials have been carried out to see how well complementary therapies work for people with cancer. Some trials are still in progress. But we need more studies to help us develop our knowledge about the best way to use complementary therapies.

What alternative therapies are

Unlike complementary therapies, alternative therapies are used instead of conventional medical treatment. People with cancer have various reasons for wanting to try alternative therapies. Some people may not start conventional treatment and may choose to use an alternative therapy instead. Some people might stop conventional cancer treatment and switch to an alternative therapy.

Some alternative therapists may claim to be able to cure your cancer with their treatments, even if conventional medical treatments haven't been able to do so. Or a therapist may say that conventional cancer treatments are harmful. A trustworthy therapist with a good reputation won't claim this.

There is no scientific or medical evidence to show that alternative therapies can cure cancer. Some alternative therapies are unsafe

and can cause harmful side-effects or they may interfere with your conventional medical treatment. Giving up your conventional cancer treatment could reduce your chance of curing or controlling your cancer.

Some alternative therapies are very cleverly promoted so that people reading about them think that they work very well. But the claims are not supported by scientific evidence and they may unfortunately give some people false hope.

Examples of alternative cancer therapies include:

⇨ Laetrile

⇨ Gerson therapy

⇨ Shark cartilage.

Other terms used to describe complementary and alternative therapies

There are several different terms commonly used to describe complementary or alternative therapies. If you are not familiar with them, it can be confusing. You may see therapies described as:

Unconventional therapies

This generally means treatments that aren't normally used by doctors to treat cancer. In other words, any treatment that is not thought of as part of conventional medicine.

Health professionals working in cancer care are becoming more aware of the differences between complementary therapies and alternative therapies. And they know how important it is to make a distinction between the two terms. Now most doctors and nurses describe therapies as either complementary or alternative, rather than unconventional.

CAM (Complementary and Alternative Medicine)

CAM is a term which covers both complementary and alternative medical therapies.

Integrated healthcare or integrated medicine

These terms are generally used to describe the use of conventional medicine and complementary therapies together. The terms are commonly used in the USA but are becoming more widely used in the UK. In cancer care, integrated medicine usually includes making sure that you have access to:

⇨ Conventional medical treatments

⇨ Different types of complementary therapies such as massage, reflexology, relaxation, herbal medicine and acupuncture

⇨ Counselling services and support groups

⇨ Up-to-date information about your cancer and its treatment.

Traditional medicine

Health professionals usually use the term 'traditional medicine' to mean a therapy or health practice that has developed over centuries within a particular culture. It is usually formed around a particular belief system. This term can be confusing because in the western part of the world conventional medicine could be considered to be a traditional medicine. But we don't usually use the term traditional medicine in this way. We usually mean it to refer to therapies or treatments that developed in the eastern part of the world such as:

⇨ Ayurvedic medicine

⇨ Traditional Chinese medicine.

What conventional medicine means

Conventional medicine is the sort of medicine and treatment your doctor would usually use to treat your cancer. You may also hear this called orthodox medical treatment. The most common treatments include:

⇨ Chemotherapy

⇨ Radiotherapy

⇨ Surgery

⇨ Biological therapies

⇨ Hormone therapy.

All conventional cancer treatments are tested thoroughly in clinical trials to prove that they work for specific types of cancer. The aim of treatment is to kill or remove, and hopefully cure, the cancer. Or if it is not curable the aim may be to control the cancer for as long as possible. Your doctor will discuss with you how likely the treatment is to help in your particular situation.

Nearly half of all conventional medicines or drugs are developed from plants or other natural substances. As conventional drugs, they are tested and used in a controlled way.

Clinical trials are carried out to:

⇨ Make sure that conventional treatments work

⇨ Make sure we know what the side effects are

⇨ Show us that the benefits of a treatment for cancer outweigh any risks.

31 December 2012

⇨ The above information is reprinted with kind permission from Cancer Research UK. Please visit www.cancerresearchuk.org for further information.

© Cancer Research UK 2014

How to choose a CAM practitioner

If you have decided to use a complementary or alternative medicine (CAM), you'll need to find a practitioner who will carry out the treatment in a way that is suitable for you.

If you think you may have a health condition, first see your GP. Do not use a visit to a CAMs practitioner as a substitute for a visit to a GP.

When you're deciding whether or not to use a CAM, the first step is to learn as much as possible about the treatment.

You should find out:

⇨ What is the evidence that this treatment is safe for you to take? For example, ginseng has been associated with higher blood pressure and may be inappropriate if you already have raised blood pressure (hypertension).

⇨ If you are using the CAM to treat a health condition, what is the evidence that the treatment works for your condition?

⇨ You can learn more about evidence in *What is evidence?* (http://www.nhs.uk/Livewell/complementary-alternative-medicine/Pages/what-is-scientific-evidence.aspx).

For further advice on whether to use a CAM, talk to your GP. It's particularly important to talk to your GP if you have a pre-existing health condition or are pregnant. Some CAMs may interact with medicines that you are taking.

Finding a practitioner

If you've learned about a particular CAM and you want to use it, you'll need to find a practitioner.

Various organisations exist that can help you to do this.

Osteopathy and chiropractic

Currently, practitioners of two CAMs are regulated in the same way as practitioners of conventional medicine. These are osteopathy and chiropractic. This regulation is called statutory professional regulation.

These regulatory bodies can help you find a registered practitioner, but they do not 'recommend' particular registered practitioners.

You can use the website of the General Osteopathic Council to find a registered osteopath near you, or check if someone offering osteopathic services is registered.

You can use the website of the General Chiropractic Council to find a registered chiropractor near you or check if someone offering chiropractic services is registered.

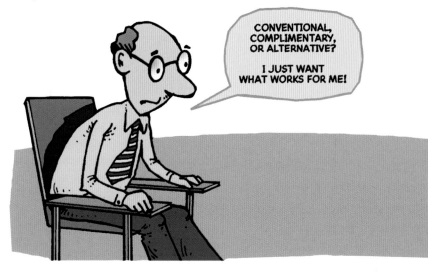

CONVENTIONAL, COMPLIMENTARY, OR ALTERNATIVE?

I JUST WANT WHAT WORKS FOR ME!

Never use an unregistered practitioner of osteopathy or chiropractic.

Other complementary and alternative treatments

In the UK, there is currently no statutory professional regulation of any other CAMs practitioners.

This means that some practitioners of these treatments may have no or limited formal training or experience. To find out more about this see *How CAM is regulated* (http://www.nhs.uk/Livewell/complementary-alternative-medicine/Pages/complementary-alternative-medicine-CAM-regulation.aspx).

Many CAMs have voluntary registers (some of which are approved by the Professional Standards Authority (PSA) for Health and Social Care) or professional associations that practitioners can join if they choose.

Organisations with PSA-accredited voluntary registers include:

⇨ Complementary & Natural Healthcare Council

⇨ British Acupuncture Council.

The websites of such organisations list practitioners who have registered with them across a wide range of therapies, such as aromatherapy, acupuncture, massage therapy and the Alexander technique.

Other professional associations hold membership lists or registers of practitioners of specific CAMs. Examples include:

⇨ British Homeopathic Association

⇨ The Reiki Association

⇨ Register of Chinese Herbal Medicine.

Health and safety in acupuncture

Although there is no statutory regulation of acupuncture, anyone practicing acupuncture must register with their local authority (council) for health and safety reasons.

This is because of the risk of contracting blood-borne diseases from piercing the skin with acupuncture needles. These rules also cover tattooing and cosmetic piercings.

The local authority must also ensure that it has byelaws that govern the cleanliness of the acupuncture premises, practitioners, instruments, materials and equipment. Disposable needles are recommended.

Once you have found a practitioner

If you have found specific practitioners, you should ask some key questions before you begin treatment.

It's a good idea to approach more than one practitioner so that you can compare them for training and experience, as well as compare the service they offer and the cost.

Ask for proof

Any good practitioner should be happy to answer questions about their qualifications and experience. You should also consider asking for:

⇨ documentary proof of their qualifications

⇨ documentary proof that they are a member of their statutory regulatory body, a voluntary register or a professional association

⇨ documentary proof that they are insured

⇨ written references.

Questions to ask

Once you are satisfied on the above, ask key questions on the service provided by the practitioner. This can help prevent problems later on.

What is the cost of treatment?

If, in addition to appointments, there are treatments that you must buy – for example, homeopathic remedies – what will they cost? Is there a charge for cancelling an appointment? Some of the organisations that support CAM practitioners may be able to give you an idea of the typical cost of treatment.

How long will the CAM treatment last?

This will vary depending on individual circumstances, but your practitioner should be able to give an estimate. The practitioner should provide you with a treatment plan that includes the number of treatments necessary to determine whether the treatment is helping. You should not have to commit to long stretches of treatment in advance, and you should discuss whether you will be asked to pay in advance of sessions.

Are there any people who should not use this treatment?

If you are pregnant or have a health condition, talk to your GP too.

What side effects might the treatment cause?

For example, are you likely to feel tired or uncomfortable afterwards? This may impact on your plans for the rest of the day and on how you will get home.

Is there anything you should do to prepare for treatment?

What system does the practitioner have for dealing with complaints about their treatment or service?

23 November 2012

⇨ The above information is reprinted with kind permission from NHS Choices. Please visit www.nhs.uk for further information.

Complementary and alternative medicine (CAM) plays an important role in healthcare in Europe – but too little is known about it

Researchers of the EU project CAMbrella call for a coordinated approach in a 'Roadmap for European CAM research'.

The scientists of CAMbrella, an EU-funded pan-European research network for CAM, today present the findings of their three years' work. They confirm that CAM is a much neglected area of research and that knowledge, provision and handling of CAM differs greatly in the different countries of Europe. Europe lags behind North America, Asia and Australia in its approach to CAM and there is an urgent need for a centralised and coordinated effort to enhance the knowledge about this field. The researchers called for a coordinated European approach, presenting a 'Roadmap for European CAM research'.

CAM is in high demand by the citizens of Europe: as many as half of all citizens in Europe use complementary and alternative medicine for their healthcare needs; speaking at the final conference in Brussels today, project coordinator Dr Wolfgang Weidenhammer, centre for CAM research at the TU Munich, said: 'Citizens are the driver for the use of CAM. Their needs and views on CAM are a key priority and their interests must be investigated and addressed in future CAM research.'

There are more than 150,000 registered medical doctors with additional CAM certification in Europe and more than 180,000 registered and certified non-medical CAM practitioners, meaning up to 65 CAM providers per 100,000 inhabitants compared to the EU figures of 95 general medical practitioners per 100,000 inhabitants. However, regulation of and education in CAM is different in each of the 39 European countries. Speaking at the conference, Prof. Vinjar Fonnebo, director of the Norwegian Institute for CAM research at the University of Tromso said: 'The current EU regulation and education chaos for CAM provision makes it impossible for health professionals to give safety and security to their patients and clients.'

Substantial lack of data about CAM

To date, there has been no thorough investigation of this field of health care in Europe. There is almost no knowledge about the prevalence of CAM use by European citizens and patients. In most European countries, there has been no research into the needs of citizens regarding CAM provision and nothing much is known about the providers' concerns.

What is CAM and what do people use it for?

CAM is an umbrella term for popular treatment strategies mostly outside conventional medicine. Practices such as herbal medicine, homeopathy, manual therapy (massage, osteopathy and reflexology), acupuncture, anthroposophic medicine or naturopathy are applied in the care of chronic conditions, disease prevention and health management. Herbal medicine is the most frequently reported CAM practice, and musculoskeletal problems the most reported conditions for the use of CAM.

The CAMbrella 'Roadmap for European CAM research'

The CAMbrella researchers call on the EU to support and implement CAM research that pays proper attention to the real world conditions of European healthcare. Professor Jarle Aarbacke, rector of University of Tromso explains, 'CAM is not part of the medicine we teach and learn in European universities – but it is nevertheless used by large numbers of patients and providers across Europe, so better we understand more about it.'

'If CAM is to be employed as part of the solution to the healthcare challenges we face in 2020, it is vital to obtain reliable information on its cost, safety and effectiveness in real world settings. CAMbrella's vision is for an evidence base which enables European citizens and policy makers to make informed decisions about CAM,' adds Prof. Dr. Benno Brinkhaus, who has led the roadmap work package, at the conference today.

CAMbrella recommends the establishment of a European research centre for CAM, allowing researchers to develop a uniform and scientific approach to CAM research, and thereby to determine the prevalence of CAM in Europe, research the most promising CAM treatments for the most common health problems such as obesity, diabetes and cancer; review patient safety, and evaluate the integration of CAM into routine healthcare treatments.

And Dr Weidenhammer sums up: 'The CAMbrella project thus plays a central role for CAM and healthcare in Europe, it all depends now on taking up the proposals and put them in action.'

29 November 2012

⇨ The above information is reprinted with kind permission from CAMbrella. Please visit www.cambrella.eu for further information.

CAM on the up as more people look for an alternative

From The Centre for the Study of Complementary Medicine, Southampton.

The last ten years has seen a marked rise in interest in complementary and alternative medicine; so much so that it is now the second largest growth industry in Europe, after IT.

Ten to 20% of the UK population visit a complementary medicine practitioner each year and between £1.5–5 billion per annum is spent on therapies or products allied to complementary medicine. Shampoos are now herbal: bath oils are now aromatherapeutic and if we follow the example of the USA, where $30 billion is spent on complementary medicine per annum, the trend will continue to grow.

Women tend to use complementary medicine more than men – but they are also more likely to go to their GP. In general, people who take care of their health and who are aware of the effect of diet on overall health will also look to complementary medicine as a means of taking responsibility for their own health. Many of those who seek out complementary medicine are wary of conventional medicine and its side effects or have found conventional medicine ineffective in dealing with long-term chronic illness. Others are using complementary medicine not because they are ill but to increase their general health and sense of well-being and as an antidote to a stressful lifestyle.

Despite the growing use of non-conventional medicine, there is still a fair amount of confusion about the different terminology, especially between alternative therapy, complementary medicine and holistic therapies. *The Which? Guide to Complementary Medicine* (Penguin Paperbacks – £9.99) defines alternative medicine as those therapies which are used in place of orthodox or conventional medicine. Complementary medicine, on the other hand, is regarded as working in conjunction with mainstream medicine.

Certainly many GPs now offer therapies as part of a patient's treatment plan and some GP practices have a counsellor or an osteopath, for example, as part of their practice team. There are also homeopathic hospitals funded by the NHS in London, Bristol, Tunbridge Wells and Glasgow and 40% of current GPs have had some training in homeopathy.

Holistic, within this context, just means treating the whole person: recognising that the mind (and spirit) can have an effect on bodily health. Holistic therapists will take longer with a patient than a GP can normally allow and they will investigate lifestyle, relationships, diet, occupation, etc., so as to take the various facets of the patient into account when treating their illness.

In everyday life, the different terms are actually used very loosely and certainly not exclusively. Many people use the term 'alternative' to refer to the more 'hippy' therapies or Eastern lifestyle therapies but I doubt that those many thousands of people who practise yoga or visit a Reiki practitioner engage in these activities instead of going to their GP.

One means of separating the terms is by noting that there is a growing body of 'scientific' evidence to support the benefits of the mainstream complementary therapies such as acupuncture, homeopathy, osteopathy and herbalism, whereas much of the evidence for the other therapies is anecdotal.

Many people would argue that because of the holistic nature of complementary medicine, the usual scientific tests are too unsophisticated to aid our understanding of what helps us get better. In this context, the latest *British Medical Journal* report on the efficacy of butterbur in treating hay fever is very interesting. The scientists' conclusions are that butterbur works as well as conventional medicines and without drowsiness, but they are forced to admit that they are unsure quite how it works and whether its active ingredients react adversely with conventional medicines.

It is certainly wise to check the qualifications of any practitioner before a consultation and to ensure that they are insured to practice. Also, if a therapist is a member of a professional body, they will have to maintain the standards and ethics of that body and are more likely to refer your problem on if they feel that they are out of their depth. Doctors, physiotherapists and osteopaths, for example, have to belong to a regulatory body, but for other therapists there is very little legislation to govern their actions or protect their patients. Those safety issues aside, choosing a therapist or indeed a therapy, is often a matter for the individual and many recommendations are by word of mouth. If you do not have good information on available services, locally, the British Complementary Medicine Association, telephone 0845 345 5977 can provide information on who is registered with them and advice on the different types of therapies, and Yellow Pages or the Internet will have listings of therapists, with their appropriate qualifications.

If you have private health insurance that covers complementary therapies, the insurers usually require that the practitioner holds a certain level of qualification and that you are referred by your GP. So alerting your GP to your intention can be a matter of financial importance as well as a matter of courtesy, however 'alternative' you go.

⇨ The above information is reprinted with kind permission from What Medicine? Please visit www.whatmedicine.co.uk for further information.

© What Medicine? 2014

Has regulation finally caught up with homeopathy in the UK?

Homeopaths in the UK are about to find out what it's like to be properly regulated... and they don't like it. Consolidation of existing regulations by the Medicines and Healthcare products Regulatory Agency (MHRA) will come into force in July 2012 despite a vigorous campaign by supporters of homeopathy. While the details of the regulations take a little effort to get your head around, there are a couple of good summaries of the situation, particularly on the UK Parliament website.

Consolidation of the regulations in this way does nothing more dramatic than bring homeopathy products under the same restrictions as other products that make therapeutic claims.

This is a big problem for homeopaths because the situation in the UK is that there are only five appropriately qualified pharmacies under the regulations which can dispense the four dozen or so formally registered potions that can be legally sold.

All other homeopathic prescribing and supply not involving a face-to-face consultation with a registered homeopath will be unlawful after 1 July 2012.

The thousands of unregistered homeopathic preparations that are not included in the regulations (equivalent to our Therapeutic Good Administration (TGA) registered products) will no longer be legal for sale. Even for the handful of legal preparations, supply without a face-to-face consultation will cease. All online sales will be illegal, and even phone ordering will have to cease.

Note that all this has occurred without the law being changed. The implication is that since the Medicines Act was introduced in 1969, it has never been properly enforced with regard to these products. The MHRA has been very firm in responding to the campaign against the changes, and has emphasised that this is not a new law, or even an amendment to existing laws. It is merely a decision to treat all therapeutic products the same, removing the anomalous status of fanciful homeopathic remedies like Dolphin Sonar or Berlin Wall that have existed for over 40 years.

Homeopaths affected by the new interpretation of the Medicines Act really have no recourse with legislation either, as MHRA has made it clear that any change to existing UK law to allow sale of these products would directly contravene EU law. This would require a massive legal and political process that would take years, and require political will that does not exist for any other issue short of national security issues.

The regulatory measures will of course only succeed if they are enforced. It is heartening to those of us who value consumer protection that the privileged position of homeopathic remedies is being ended, but one fears the MHRA may be in a similar position to our own TGA. Open flouting of minimal regulations without fear of meaningful sanction such as happens here could be possible. Companies in Australia that run afoul of regulations can afford to take a calculated risk that their profits will far outweigh any puny attempts by TGA to bring them to book. Much like choosing to cop a parking fine occasionally because paying for car parking may work out more expensive if done regularly.

Supporters of homeopathy in Australia may call for statutory regulation of Alt Med professions but I must say this is the type of evidence-based, low-cost regulatory reform that makes most sense. Homeopathy as such has not been made illegal. It has just been stopped from fleecing consumers by selling unregulated products and making unfounded claims about them.

27 June 2012

⇨ The above information is reprinted with kind permission from The Conversation. Please visit www.theconversation.com for further information.

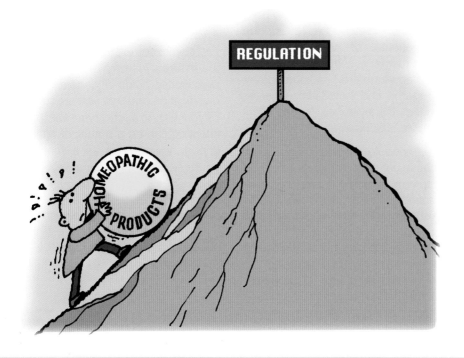

EU herbal medicines legislation fails again

Broken regulations affecting herbal products in the European Union (EU) and herbal practitioners in the UK are in the news again. The European Medicines Agency (EMA) has just published its latest, damning 'school report' on the EU's Traditional Herbal Medicinal Products Directive (THMPD). Coupled with the stalling of UK Government plans to bring in statutory regulation of herbalists, the future for herbalism remains manifestly unsettled.

New traditional use registrations down year-on-year

The latest EMA report on the THMPD covers the period up to and including 31 December 2012, in addition to the data in its two previous reports. A total of 264 new traditional use registrations (TURs) were granted EU-wide to herbal medicinal products in 2012 (Figure 1), bringing the grand total to 1,015 (673 single-herb, 342 polyherbal) since the THMPD became law on 30 April 2004.

Of these 264 new TURs, 163 were for single-herb products and 101 for polyherbal products, the first time since the THMPD became operative that new TURs have dropped – by a whopping 29.6% – year-on-year. We appear to have passed 'peak TUR'.

Well-established use authorisations stable

Marketing authorisations granted under the well-established use (WEU) provisions of Directive 2001/83/EC have remained consistent (Figure 2), with 82 in total for 2012 – 59 for single-herb products, 23 for polyherbal formulations – up by nine (12.3%) compared with 2011. Because of their increased rigour relative to the already strict THMPD, WEU marketing authorisations are only accessible to the largest and best-funded companies. And with the number of new TURs in steep decline, the smaller companies that are the lifeblood of the herbal industry are being shut out more than ever.

Not a very 'traditional' directive

A closer look at the 342 polyherbal TUR products (Figure 3) shows that the vast majority (n=246; 71.9%) consist of two to four herbal components. There are 67 (19.5%) products containing five to nine components, a drop in percentage terms compared with 2011 [http://anh-europe.org/news/european-medicines-agency-releases-second-report-on-eu-herbal-directive]. In no way does this situation accurately reflect the practise of any long-standing herbal tradition, since formulae in the Western tradition commonly contain five to ten herbs and those used by Indian Ayurveda and traditional Chinese medicine (TCM) often contain 12 or more. Ayurvedic chyawanprash may contain up to 80 herbs, and commonly includes 40–50 ingredients!

The incredible shrinking traditions

The pharmacopoeias of just Western herbal medicine, Ayurveda and TCM include up to 1,500 different plant species. By contrast, after nearly a decade of operation, the THMPD's simplified registration scheme has allowed a total of 133 herbal species through its doors, very few of which are associated exclusively with non-European traditions. The list of approved indications for TUR herbal products is similarly brief, consisting of a mere 14 therapeutic areas.

The THMPD: not fit for purpose!

There's no need for anyone to make a case against the THMPD based on the text of the legislation and its theoretical impact on the herbal products market, because the EMA's own figures utterly condemn the herbal directive. There is almost zero chances that common sense will prevail and EU regulators, supported by Member States, will see sense and repeal the law. The only practical way of fixing the THMPD, we believe, is through a favourable judgement at the European Court of Justice – which is what our legal challenge is all about.

Figure 1. Number of TURs granted each year under the THMPD (2004 until 31 December 2012; total 1,015).

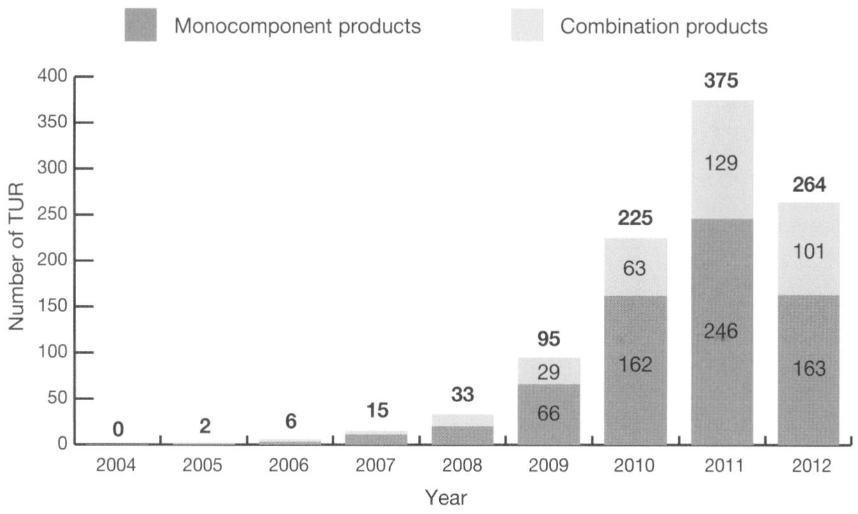

Source: Uptake of the traditional use registration scheme and implementation of the provisions of Directive 2004/24/EC in EU Member States, 17 June 2014, European Medicines Agency.

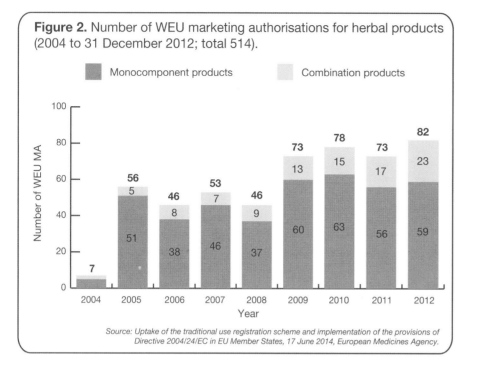

Figure 2. Number of WEU marketing authorisations for herbal products (2004 to 31 December 2012; total 514).

Monocomponent products   Combination products

Source: Uptake of the traditional use registration scheme and implementation of the provisions of Directive 2004/24/EC in EU Member States, 17 June 2014, European Medicines Agency.

UK herbalists in the long grass

Yesterday, on Tuesday 9 July, UK Member of Parliament David Tredinnick hosted a debate on statutory regulation (SR) of the country's herbalists. Many people in the UK are wondering what their government is up to, after it promised SR in 2011 and then did precisely nothing. The minister responsible for herbal medicine policy, Dr Dan Poulter, attended the debate, and his comments provided the first developments in quite some time.

In short, the Government is kicking the entire issue into the long grass using the time-honoured politician's technique of the infinite consultation. After literally decades of meetings, consultations, working groups, committees and focus groups to get us to this point, Dr Poulter proposed... another working group to discuss the 'complex' issues raised by SR.

Polish problems

Once again, Dr Poulter is using as justification a recent judgement on a Polish case in the European Court of Justice (ECJ) that reveals Poland broke the law by importing cheap, unlicensed medicines – even though the imports were identical in terms of active substance, dose and form. The ECJ reached this

conclusion because the imported medicines had not been granted a marketing authorisation according to EU medicines law. Dr Poulter's comments on the Polish case confirm the statement made by Lord Pearson of Rannoch in a House of Lords debate on SR held on 24 April.

This is strange logic indeed, since SR would allow the UK to comply with EU medicines law whereas Poland was deliberately flouting it, albeit with some justification. But it's heartening at least to know that the UK Government thinks little of the argument proposed by skeptics

like Lord Taverne, that SR would confer spurious respectability on a 'quack' profession.

We'll be there!

Although we're not convinced of the need for yet more discussions on this issue, we can confirm that we will be directly involved in them and we'll keep you posted on developments. Along with others involved in the recent SR campaign, such as the European Herbal & Traditional Medicine Practitioners Association, we have been working hard behind the scenes to get to this point – so it's a shame that none of these organisations were mentioned during yesterday's debate.

EU herbal medicines legislation, then: it's a complete mess. The sooner we can get into court and sort it out, the better – we look forward to your support!

10 July 2013

⇨ The above information is reprinted with kind permission from Alliance for Natural Health Europe. Please visit www. anh-europe.org for further information.

© *Alliance for Natural Health Europe 2014*

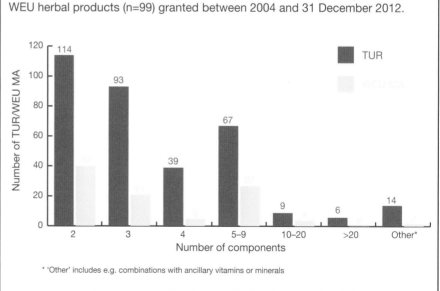

Figure 3. Number of herbal components in polyherbal TUR (n=342) and WEU herbal products (n=99) granted between 2004 and 31 December 2012.

* 'Other' includes e.g. combinations with ancillary vitamins or minerals

Source: Uptake of the traditional use registration scheme and implementation of the provisions of Directive 2004/24/EC in EU Member States, 17 June 2014, European Medicines Agency.

Regulation of herbal medicines – Commons Library Standard Note

By Dr Sarah Barber

This Note outlines the historical regulation of herbal medicines in the UK, regulatory changes due to the EU Directive on Traditional Herbal Medicinal Products, and proposals to introduce statutory registration of herbal practitioners.

Herbal remedies for human use have for some time been regarded as medicines under UK legislation, in principle subject to the same licensing procedures as pharmaceuticals. In particular, efficacy requirements have been difficult to meet and so most EU Member States developed various pragmatic arrangements to tackle this. In the UK herbal remedies have historically been exempted from licensing.

A review of herbal regulation at EU level was prompted by safety concerns and the need for market harmonisation of various national herbal regulatory regimes.

The Directive on Traditional Herbal Medicinal Products (Directive 2004/24/EC) replaces most existing member state regulations and creates a unified licensing system for traditional herbal medicine products (in use for at least 30 years, of which 15 must usually have been in the EU). The Directive came into full effect on 30 April 2011.

The Directive applies to manufactured herbal medicinal products sold over the counter, prohibiting the continued sale of unlicensed products. This note will outline the conditions in which herbal medicines can now be sold in the UK.

The Directive has met with some opposition from suppliers and users of herbal medicines. Objections include perceived disproportionate costs of regulatory compliance and the difficulty some non-European herbal traditions may have in meeting the requirement. There are concerns this will result in threatening the viability of businesses and a reduction in consumer choice.

In February 2011, a statutory regulation scheme for herbal practitioners was proposed which would allow prescribing of unlicensed preparations by registered herbalists under a clause in the 2001 Medicines Directive. It was planned that this scheme would come into force in 2012. In July this year, the Under Secretary of State for Health, Dr Daniel Poulter highlighted issues which have made the introduction of the scheme difficult. He announced the setting up of a working group to further consider evidence and options. It will meet for the first time in early 2014.

12 February 2014

⇨ The above information contains Parliamentary information licensed under the Open Parliament Licence v1.0. Please visit www.parliament.co.uk for further information.

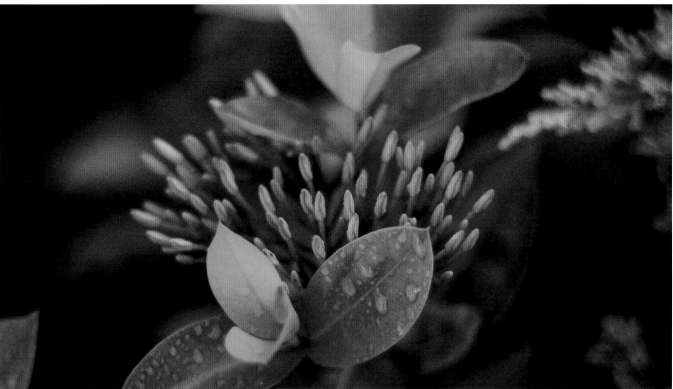

How CAM is regulated

The practise of conventional medicine is regulated by special laws that ensure that practitioners are properly qualified, and adhere to certain standards or codes of practice.

This is called statutory professional regulation. Professionals of two complementary and alternative treatments – osteopathy and chiropractic – are regulated in the same way. But there is no statutory professional regulation of any other complementary and alternative medicine (CAM) practitioners.

Most complementary and alternative medicine practitioners are not regulated by professional statutory regulation. This means it is up to you to find out whether your practitioner has qualifications, and will conduct treatment in a way that is acceptable to you.

Many complementary and alternative medicines have professional associations and/or voluntary registers, which practitioners can join if they choose. Usually, these associations or registers demand that practitioners hold certain qualifications, and agree to practise to a certain standard. However, in these cases there is no legal requirement that practitioners join an association or register before they start to practise.

Regulation of complementary and alternative medicine

Currently, practitioners of two complementary and alternative medicines are regulated in the same way as practitioners of conventional medicine. They are osteopathy and chiropractic. This regulation is called statutory professional regulation.

This regulation ensures that registered practitioners of osteopathy and chiropractic are properly qualified, and that they practise in a way that is safe and ethical, following the standards and codes set by their professional regulators.

These regulatory bodies can help you to find a registered practitioner, but they do not 'recommend' particular registered practitioners.

⇨ All osteopaths must be registered with the General Osteopathic Council. It is illegal to call yourself an osteopath, or offer services as a registered osteopath, without registration. You can learn more, and find a registered osteopath near you, at the website of the General Osteopathic Council.

⇨ All chiropractors must be registered with the General Chiropractic Council. It is illegal to call yourself a chiropractor, or offer services as a registered chiropractor, without registration. You can learn more, and find a registered chiropractor, at the website of the General Chiropractic Council.

Regulation exists to protect patient safety: it does not by itself mean that there is scientific evidence that a treatment is effective. To find out whether a treatment is effective, you need to learn more about the evidence for that treatment.

Unregulated complementary and alternative medicines

In the UK, there is currently no statutory professional regulation of any other complementary and alternative medicine practitioners.

This means, for example, that anyone in the UK can legally call themselves a homeopath and practise homeopathy on patients, even if they have no training or experience. These practitioners are not legally required to adhere to any standards of practice. If you have a complaint about treatment you have received from a homeopath, you have no special legal rights beyond normal civil and criminal law.

The same applies to all other complementary and alternative medicines, except osteopathy and chiropractic (see above). This means that some practitioners of these treatments may have no or limited formal training or experience.

If you want to use an unregulated complementary or alternative medicine, it's up to you to find a practitioner who will practise in a way that is acceptable to you.

Some regulated practitioners of conventional medicine also practise unregulated CAMs. For example, the Faculty of Homeopathy is a voluntary organisation for statutorily regulated health professionals, such as GPs, who also practise homeopathy. The organisations who regulate these professionals do not regulate their CAM practice, but would investigate concerns that relate to the professional conduct of their registered practitioner.

Voluntary registers

In the case of many complementary and alternative medicines there are professional associations or voluntary registers that practitioners can choose to join.

Typically, practitioners can only join these associations or registers if they hold certain qualifications, and agree to adhere to certain standards of practice. However, there is no legal requirement to join and practitioners can still offer services without being a member of any organisation.

If you want to use a complementary and alternative medicine where practitioners are not regulated by professional statutory regulation, you should make use of professional bodies or voluntary registers, where they exist, to help you find a practitioner.

You may want to check what arrangements there are for complaining about a practitioner. For example, does the association or register accept complaints, and what action will they take if you have concerns about your treatment?

23 November 2012

⇨ The above information is reprinted with kind permission from NHS Choices. Please visit www.nhs.uk for further information.

UK launches new programme to reduce demand for tiger parts

The UK Government today announced its support for a programme to protect and recover wild tigers by reducing the demand for their bones and other body parts.

The commitment is part of the UK Government's ongoing support for the Global Tiger Recovery Program (GTRP), endorsed by all 13 tiger range countries at the 'Tiger Summit' held in St Petersburg in 2010 and was made ahead of the London Conference on Illegal Wildlife Trade currently taking place and hosted by UK Foreign Secretary William Hague.

'Today's conference is about bringing together world leaders to find real answers to the devastation of wildlife crime. This is something that brings untold misery to people across Africa, and feeds regional and international instability. Above all though, it is a terrible act that endangers species and threatens entire ecosystems. That is why this government is funding TRAFFIC to help reduce demand for tiger products. I hope that the conference, along with the excellent work being done by TRAFFIC, will encourage others to protect this beautiful animal before it is too late,' said the UK Government's Foreign & Commonwealth Office Minister for Africa, Mark Simmonds.

Demand for tiger parts and derivatives continues to drive poaching of tigers and fuels an increasingly sophisticated network of illegal wildlife trafficking in the 13 tiger range countries.

The announcement came as new figures and photographs were released highlighting the critical situation facing wild tigers from poaching activities. According to new research carried out by TRAFFIC, parts of 1,537 tigers have been seized in illegal trade across 13 tiger range countries in the 14 years between 2000 and 2013. The figures equates to 110 tiger parts trafficked per year, or two per week.

The startling figures were announced as new photographs of poachers attempting to sell tiger bones were released. The images were taken last month in Labuhanbatu province, Sumatra, Indonesia by tiger conservationists posing as buyers.

The poachers claimed to have snared and sold the bones and other body parts of tigers on three occasions since 2012. They told the undercover researchers the skin, teeth and claws were sold separately as they were more valuable.

'The unremitting poaching pressure is steadily but relentlessly pushing the Sumatran and other wild tiger populations towards the same fate as those in Bali and Java,' said Steven Broad, Executive Director of TRAFFIC.

'As TRAFFIC's latest research and these photographs from Indonesia demonstrate, there is still some way to go to achieving the critical first step to accomplish the overall GTRP goal of doubling the number of wild tigers by 2022 – that of securing zero poaching of wild tigers.'

Across Asia, wild tiger numbers have plummeted from an estimated 100,000 animals at the turn of the 20th century to as few as 3,200 today.

In Indonesia there are believed to be fewer than 500 wild tigers left, all on the island of Sumatra. Tigers became extinct on the Indonesian islands of Bali in the 1940s and Java in the 1970s.

The seed money for this programme to address demand is being administered through a grant made to TRAFFIC from the GTRP Multi-Donor Trust Fund. This fund, administered by the World Bank, provides global support on the ground for the GTRP. It helps fill financing gaps with pooled funding from governmental, corporate and private donors. The UK Government is the initial contributor to the fund. TRAFFIC's partners in this project include WildAid, WWF and the Zoological Society of London.

'As tiger range countries have stepped up national efforts and made measurable progress in implementing the Global Tiger Recovery Program since the Tiger Summit in 2010, demand reduction is an element of global support that has taken time to get off the ground,' said Andrey Kushlin, Program Manager, Global Tiger Initiative, World Bank.

'By drawing on the body of work that has already been done on behaviour change and demand reduction, TRAFFIC and other partners help the efforts of the tiger range countries in finally breathing life into demand reduction work of the GTRP, supported by this Multi Donor Trust fund.

'The London Conference is also a great opportunity for partners and donors to expand their support for these aspects of tiger conservation.'

Guest author:

Dr Richard Thomas is the Global Communications Co-ordinator working with TRAFFIC to monitor and combat the illegal wildlife trade.

12 February 2014

⇨ The above information is reprinted with kind permission from Dr Richard Thomas/ TRAFFIC. Please visit www.traffic.org for further information.

About complementary medicines

Complementary and alternative medicines are treatments that fall outside of mainstream healthcare.

These medicines and treatments range from acupuncture and homeopathy to aromatherapy, meditation and colonic irrigation.

There is no universally agreed definition of complementary and alternative medicine (CAM).

The information that tells whether a healthcare treatment is safe and effective is called evidence. You can use evidence to help you decide whether you want to use a CAM. Detailed information on many complementary and alternative treatments can be found listed on the NHS website in the Health A-Z index.

Some complementary and alternative medicines or treatments are based on principles and an evidence base that are not recognised by the majority of independent scientists.

The availability of complementary and alternative treatments on the NHS is limited. Some, such as acupuncture, may be offered by the NHS in some circumstances.

'Alternative' and 'complementary' defined

Although 'complementary and alternative' is often used as a single category, it can be useful to make a distinction between complementary and alternative medicine.

This distinction is about two different ways of using these treatments:

⇨ Treatments are sometimes used to provide an experience that is pleasant in itself. This can include use alongside conventional treatments, to help a patient cope with a health condition. When used this way the treatment is not intended as an alternative to conventional treatment. The US National Center for Complementary and Alternative Medicine (NCCAM) says that use of treatments in this way can be called complementary medicine.

⇨ Treatments are sometimes used instead of conventional medicine, with the intention of treating or curing a health condition. The NCCAM says that use of treatments in this way can be called alternative medicine.

There can be overlap between these two categories. For example, aromatherapy may sometimes be used as a complementary treatment, and in other circumstances is used as an alternative treatment.

A number of complementary and alternative treatments are typically used with the intention of treating or curing a health condition. Examples include:

⇨ homeopathy

⇨ acupuncture

⇨ osteopathy

⇨ chiropractic

⇨ herbalism.

Evidence and complementary or alternative treatments

Given the extremely wide range of complementary and alternative medicines on offer, how can we decide whether to use one of these treatments?

To make such a decision, we need evidence on whether a treatment is safe and effective.

We also need to find out whether there is a suitable practitioner available to administer it.

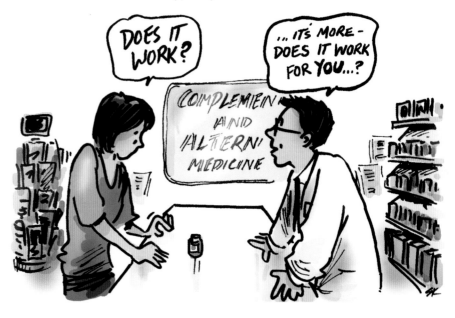

It's important to remember that when a person uses any health treatment – including a complementary or alternative medicine – and experiences an improvement, this may be due to the placebo effect.

In a few cases, certain complementary and alternative treatments have been proven to work for a limited number of health conditions. For example, there is good evidence that osteopathy, chiropractic and acupuncture work to treat persistent low back pain. These treatments are named in the NICE guidance on treatment of persistent low back pain.

Complementary and alternative medicine and the NHS

In most cases the NHS does not offer patients complementary or alternative treatments.

The National Institute for Health and Care Excellence (NICE) provides guidance to the NHS on the clinical and cost-effective use of treatments and care of patients. NICE has recommended the use of complementary and alternative medicines in a limited number of circumstances.

For example:

⇨ the Alexander technique for Parkinson's disease

⇨ ginger and acupressure for reducing morning sickness

⇨ acupuncture and manual therapy, including spinal manipulation, spinal mobilisation and massage for persistent low back pain.

NICE bases its recommendations on the available scientific evidence for the clinical and cost-effectiveness of treatments.

23 November 2012

⇨ The above information is reprinted with kind permission from NHS Choices. Please visit www.nhs.uk for further information.

© NHS Choices 2014

The cost of complementary and alternative therapies

The cost of using complementary therapies

Many cancer wards, units and hospitals in the UK offer complementary therapies to patients free of charge. You might be offered a set number of treatments free, but have to pay for any further treatment after that. This is not always the case but it is worth asking. You may also be able to have some therapies free, or at a cheaper rate, through your GP. Costs vary depending on the individual therapy.

Several independent cancer support centres provide various complementary therapies alongside conventional cancer treatments. Depending on the organisation, you may be able to have a single treatment, weekly treatments or go to the centre daily for a few days, for a complementary therapy programme that suits you. You may have to pay for the treatments you have, but there is sometimes an opportunity to pay less than the standard rate, and some centres won't charge you at all. Look at our complementary therapy organisations page for a list of centres to contact about their prices.

Some cancer support groups offer free or low cost therapies. Some charitable organisations offer free sessions of meditation, relaxation or guided visualisation. Staff at your hospital may also know of local services or you can find them on the Internet.

Private practitioners of complementary therapies can charge up to £60 or more per hour. These costs vary from place to place within the UK – for example, treatments are usually more expensive in cities.

If you are using herbal remedies, vitamins or dietary supplements the prices can vary a lot. It is important to let your doctor know if you are taking any type of herbs, vitamins or dietary supplements along with conventional cancer treatment. For information about costs of particular therapies go to the individual complementary therapies section and click on the type of therapy you are interested in.

The cost of using alternative therapies

Many alternative therapies are expensive. Some therapies might only cost a few pounds a month, but others may set you back several hundred or more. Make sure you have thought about the ongoing cost before you start taking anything or begin any treatment. There is no scientific evidence that any alternative therapy works so it is important to talk to your doctor before deciding to use any of these therapies.

⇨ The above information is reprinted with kind permission from Cancer Research UK. Please visit www.cancerresearch.org for further information.

© Cancer Research UK 2014

Complementary and alternative therapies and dementia

There are high levels of public interest in the various complementary and alternative therapies available today. Many people with dementia, and those who care for them, are interested in using these therapies as alternatives or additions to their conventional treatments, often due to the perceived benefits that they may bring and the image of being 'safe' and 'natural'. This article explains what complementary and alternative therapies are, outlines several therapies for which there is some evidence of their effectiveness and describes how to access these treatments.

This article only addresses therapies that have an evidence base and does not cover treatments for which there is no clinical evidence of effectiveness in dementia, even if they are widely used (such as homeopathy).

What are complementary and alternative therapies?

The term 'complementary and alternative therapy' covers many diverse forms of treatment.

Complementary and alternative therapies are a broad range of treatments that are outside of conventional medicine and are used to treat or prevent illness and promote health and well-being. Practitioners of complementary therapies are not trained to diagnose disease.

The area of complementary and alternative medicine is controversial and changes regularly. Therapies that are considered 'complementary' or 'alternative' in one country may be considered conventional in another. Therapies that are currently considered alternative may become more mainstream over time, as researchers discover their effectiveness and they become integrated into mainstream healthcare practice. Some complementary and alternative therapies are now available on the NHS, although this varies from region to region.

Using complementary and alternative therapy versus conventional medicine

Complementary and alternative therapy should only be used in addition to, not instead of, conventional medicine. If you decide to use complementary and alternative therapy it is important that you continue to see your doctor and keep them informed of the treatments you are having.

Although most complementary and alternative treatments have a good safety profile they are not 100 per cent safe and there are serious safety concerns about some therapies. For example, some herbal preparations may interact harmfully with conventional drugs. It is therefore very important that your doctor knows exactly what you are taking.

Don't be nervous about telling your doctor what you are using – awareness of complementary and alternative therapy is increasing among the medical profession, and most doctors are sympathetic to its use.

How widespread is complementary and alternative therapy?

At least one in four people in England are thought to have used complementary or alternative therapy in the past year. In recent surveys, 85 per cent of medical students, 76 per cent of GPs and 69 per cent of hospital doctors have said they feel that complementary therapies should be made available on the NHS. This widespread interest helps to encourage research in the area.

One common concern is the difficulty in regulating such a varied range of treatments. Most forms of complementary and alternative therapy have one or more governing bodies, which set standards for the training and services provided and codes of conduct for practitioners.

However, these are often self-regulated and membership tends to be voluntary. A report by the House of Lords in 2000 called for more regulation, and research to investigate effectiveness and safety. However, current regulation is still patchy.

In 2008 the Department of Health funded the Prince's Foundation for Integrated Health to set up the Complementary and Natural Healthcare Council to regulate 12 alternative therapies, such as aromatherapy, reflexology and homeopathy. This may serve to improve regulation in some areas, however some commentators have argued that, as membership is not mandatory, this regulation will be of doubtful value.

Can complementary and alternative therapy be used to treat dementia?

There is little high-quality research into the treatment of dementia with complementary and alternative therapy. However, research on a number of therapies is providing some interesting preliminary results and these are described in this article. There are other types of therapies that may have potential but as there is currently no evidence about their effectiveness, they are not listed here. Only you can decide whether you should try complementary and alternative therapy, but by following the information in this article you can make an informed decision.

The symptoms of dementia are numerous and change over time, but most types of dementia have some symptoms in common. If you are thinking about which complementary or alternative therapy may be most suitable, it is important to consider which specific symptoms you want to treat. The aims of treatment range from improving memory to providing relaxation.

How can I get access to complementary and alternative therapy?

The first person to speak to about accessing complementary and alternative therapy is your doctor. They may be able to tell you about the evidence, refer you through the NHS or offer advice on good practitioners in your area.

What should I look for in a practitioner?

It is advisable to find a practitioner who is registered with a governing body. It is also vital that you trust and feel comfortable with the person, as the therapeutic relationship forms an important part of complementary and alternative therapy. At the first meeting, you should ask:

⇨ what the treatment will involve

⇨ the frequency and number of visits that the treatment is likely to require

⇨ the cost of the treatment

⇨ the results you can expect to receive from the treatment

⇨ the risks of the treatment.

A good practitioner should encourage continued care with your doctor and may even liaise with them. They should also have a realistic attitude towards the therapy. For example, they should talk through the likelihood of the treatment having no effect, or possible side-effects, as well as potential benefits. Make sure you tell them about any conventional medications you are taking.

Specific treatments

The remainder of this article looks at a range of therapies, listed in alphabetical order, which may be effective in addressing certain symptoms associated with dementia.

Acupuncture

Acupuncture originated in China and views health disorders as resulting from imbalances in the flow of energy ('chi' or 'qi', pronounced 'chee') around the body. Acupuncture is said to unblock the energy pathways ('meridians') to restore functioning.

Practitioners insert very fine needles into the skin to produce the therapeutic effect.

As acupuncture has grown more popular in the West, theories about it based on Western models of medicine have developed. For example, some practitioners believe that it reduces local muscle tension, or that it affects the way the body reacts to pain. Both traditional and more modern forms of acupuncture are practised in the UK.

A number of studies have addressed the use of acupuncture for treating Alzheimer's disease and vascular dementia, and for associated mental problems, such as depression and insomnia. These studies all report positive effects, but they are generally not very well conducted, and better studies are needed to confirm these preliminary findings.

For practitioners of more traditional forms of acupuncture, contact the British Acupuncture Council. Alternatively, you may consider seeing an acupuncturist who is also a doctor (contact the British Medical Acupuncture Society) or chartered physiotherapist (contact the Acupuncture Association of Chartered Physiotherapists).

Aromatherapy

Aromatherapy is based on the theory that essential oils, derived from plants, have beneficial properties. The oils used are concentrated and it is important to use them according to instructions, for example diluting them before applying to the skin. The oils may be:

⇨ applied directly to the skin, often accompanied by massage (see 'Massage', below)

⇨ heated in an oil burner to produce a pleasant aroma

⇨ added to a bath.

There is some evidence that aromatherapy may be effective in helping people with dementia to relax and that certain oils may have the potential to improve cognition in people with Alzheimer's disease. Research has highlighted the potential benefits of aromatherapy, specifically the use of lemon balm

(*Melissa officinalis*) and lavender oil, in the treatment of Alzheimer's disease. However, there is currently insufficient evidence to state categorically whether or not it is beneficial.

Bright light therapy

Sleep disorders and disruptive nocturnal behaviour are commonly associated with dementia and present a significant clinical problem. These include a characteristic pattern of sleep disturbance referred to as 'sundowning' – increased arousal and activity, usually in the late afternoon, evening or night – which many people caring for someone with dementia find very stressful.

Bright lights have been found to be beneficial as a treatment for sleep disturbances associated with dementia. In bright light therapy, a person sits in front of a light box that provides about 30 times more light than the average office light, for a set amount of time each day. One small but well-conducted study showed promising effects of bright light therapy on restlessness and disturbed sleep for people with dementia.

A more recent study showed that using stronger general lighting in care homes improved cognition in people with dementia, enhanced their sense of night and day, enabled them to sleep better, and reduced levels of depression.

Current findings indicate that bright light therapy may benefit people with dementia, but further research is needed.

Herbal medicine

Herbal medicine uses plants to restore or maintain health. There is often variation in the quality and, therefore, the levels of the active constituents of herbal products. Since April 2011, all manufactured herbal medicines have to be registered under a new scheme, known as the Traditional Herbal Registration (THR). If you are interested in self-medication, consult your doctor first, and buy a recognised brand by a leading manufacturer.

'Phytomedicine' is a term often used to denote a more scientific approach to herbal medicine, in which products are standardised and concentrated so that they contain specified amounts of the identified active substances in the herbal products. More rigorous research is usually undertaken within this area.

Branches of herbal medicine include Western herbal medicine, Chinese traditional medicine, and kampo, a Japanese variant of Chinese medicine. The following herbs may have some effect on symptoms associated with dementia:

⇨ Choto-san – Two studies into this kampo (see above) mixture, which contains 11 medicinal plants, have found that it improved a range of symptoms in people with vascular dementia. Further research on this preparation seems justified.

⇨ Kami-Umtan-To (KUT) – This is another kampo mixture, which contains 13 different plants. A clinical trial found a slower decline in the group of people with Alzheimer's disease given this preparation.

⇨ Yizhi capsule (YZC) – Initial studies on the use of this Chinese traditional herbal medicine in patients with vascular dementia have reported positive results, although the studies were not of a high standard. Further research into this preparation seems justified, but for now the evidence is inconclusive.

⇨ Ginkgo biloba extract – Until recently it was thought that ginkgo biloba could be effective at slowing down the progression of dementia and the remedy still has its proponents. However, a study carried out in 2008 found that it has no effect and this was confirmed by reviews of a larger number of small studies.

To consult a Western herbalist, contact the National Institute of Medical Herbalists. For a Chinese herbalist contact the Register of Chinese Herbal Medicine.

Massage

There are many types of massage, but common across all of them is the hands-on manipulation of the body's soft tissue by the practitioner. Massage is often used alongside aromatherapy (see 'Aromatherapy', above).

There is much anecdotal evidence that massage can help manage symptoms associated with dementia such as anxiety, agitation and depression, but studies have not been sufficiently rigorous to provide solid proof. It does seem likely that massage interventions may well be beneficial, but further research is required.

Music therapy

Music can have a powerful effect on a person's state of mind. Music therapy uses music and other sound (such as 'white noise') to restore or improve a person's sense of well-being.

Treatment usually involves playing music or sounds that the person enjoys for up to 30 minutes in a quiet room. Someone else should be present for at least some of the time to make sure that the person with dementia is comfortable and happy with the level of sound. They can also make comments linking the sounds to the person's experiences and can encourage the person to join in with the rhythms or sing along. If there is a certain time of the day when the person with dementia becomes agitated, music therapy can be scheduled just before this time.

A review of music therapy for dementia concluded that, based on the available evidence, it is unclear whether or not music therapy is beneficial for people with dementia.

For more information about music therapy, contact the British Association for Music Therapy. Music therapists should also be registered with the Health Professions Council.

TENS

TENS (transcutaneous electrical nerve stimulation) involves applying a mild electrical current through electrodes stuck to the skin. The treatment can produce a prickling sensation but is not painful. It is often used for pain control, for example during labour.

A number of studies have suggested that the use of TENS machines may produce short-lived improvement in some of the behavioural aspects of dementia. The data available suggests that TENS may be beneficial, but the results are not yet conclusive.

TENS machines are available to buy or hire from many high-street chemists.

For information about a wide range of dementia-related topics, visit alzheimers.org.uk/factsheets.

⇨ The above information is reprinted with kind permission from Alzheimer's Society. Please visit www.alzheimers.org.uk for further information.

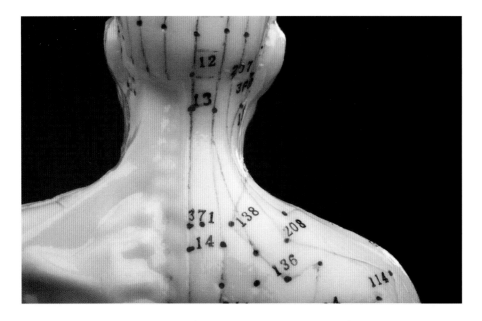

Complementary therapy gains steam in palliative care

With 90% of individuals confirming they would consider complementary therapy to help manage symptoms of terminal illness, Therapy Directory speak to two professional therapists to find out why so many people are now taking a holistic approach to help them face their biggest health challenges.

Being diagnosed with an illness that is life-threatening or that cannot be cured can be an incredibly distressing experience, and there is no right or wrong way to react to this news. Whatever those initial feelings may be, it's perfectly normal to feel a range of emotions, from shock, fear and anger through to frustration, relief and perhaps eventually, acceptance.

While a team of healthcare experts will be on hand to let individuals know what medical support is available to them, outside of traditional palliative medical care, complementary therapy is gaining steam when it comes to the management and relief of some associated physical and emotional symptoms.

According to the results of an online survey conducted by Therapy Directory – a support network of complementary therapists – a proportionate 90% of respondents said that should they be diagnosed with a terminal illness, they would consider complementary therapy to help them to deal with the symptoms [1].

So why are so many people now choosing to take a holistic approach to their health?

In a bid to understand more about the increased take up of complementary therapies in palliative care, Therapy Directory speak with two of their listed therapists for their take on the matter.

Michelle Mullis, owner of Kent Acupuncture Health, specialises in both acupuncture and aromatherapy massage and has experience of delivering both as part of palliative care.

Speaking about acupuncture treatment – in particular when delivered as an adjunctive to cancer chemotherapy treatment – Michelle explains how this natural therapy can help to reduce symptoms of nausea, fatigue, cancer pain and associated hot flushes:

'Much research supports the use of acupuncture for these symptoms. The main areas of research into acupuncture for cancer are chemotherapy-related sickness, fatigue and cancer pain. Having cancer can have a big impact on quality of life, causing distress and affecting everyday tasks, so acupuncture can help people to manage their day-to-day lives,' she explained.

Michelle is also qualified in aromatherapy treatment, another complementary therapy that she has used while working in hospice palliative care to improve quality of life. Michelle reports that as well as the physical benefits, certain oils can be incredibly soothing on an emotional level:

'Bergamot helps reduce agitation and panic and is often used in cases of depression, while Rose Otto is another oil that I use with patients as it calms anxiety and relieves tension. Ylang Ylang is also an oil that patients respond well to as this helps with fear, depression and anxiety whilst reducing the breathing pace.'

The emotional impact

Former nurse, and therapist since 2001, Emma Coleman, agrees that complementary therapies can be of benefit on both a physical and psychological level.

'In my experience as a therapist I have treated clients with cancer in numerous ways and have found that alternative approaches can vastly aid the improvement of how a sufferer feels psychologically as well as easing any physical symptoms,' she said.

Emma also explained how relaxation is the most common aim for her clients, and in an indirect way this approach can also help to alleviate the stress of close family. As a result of the client often feeling more positive and lifted after treatment, the carer or relative feels more optimistic and supported – a two-fold impact.

Finding a complementary therapist

As more people begin to lean towards a natural and holistic approach to their health, complementary therapy is being used more and more. While these types of therapy should not be viewed as a replacement for traditional medical care, what we are seeing more frequently is that when used alongside conventional medicine the benefits can be significant.

Here at Therapy Directory, we only list complementary therapists who have provided us with relevant qualifications and insurance cover, or proof of registration with a professional body – making it a great place to start for those considering introducing complementary therapy to their care plan. To start your journey to better mind, body and spirit, visit Therapy Directory today.

Notes to editors

Please note, we advise that individuals consult their GP before introducing any new therapy to their care plan. In addition, when using any complementary therapy, treatment must be tailored to individual needs and should only be carried out by an experienced practitioner.

References

[1] Results based on a survey of 41 visitors to Therapy Directory from December 2013 to January 2014.

⇨ The above information is reprinted with kind permission from Therapy Directory. Please visit www.therapy-directory.org.uk for further information.

The case for Chinese herbal medicine in the treatment of depression

More people are seeking alternatives to traditional mental health care and as a result, knowledge about the use of complementary therapies by people with mental illness is increasing – particularly for those experiencing anxiety and depression. A recent survey of women with depression revealed that there is a push for more 'natural approaches' that match with the individual's own values and beliefs. CAM (complementary and alternative medicines) are also something people turn to when they are unhappy with their existing care – users are more likely to have received mental health and primary care treatment and to be dissatisfied with their overall healthcare when compared to non-users.

Numerous systematic reviews and research papers have been published on the effects of Western herbs, such as St John's wort (Linde, Berner and Kriston Lin, 2008) in the treatment of depression, but Chinese herbs have received less attention. The aim of this article is to assess the evidence on Chinese herbal medicine treatments for depression based on previous systematic reviews of trials in the Western literature.

The supplementary review located eight trials and positive results were reported almost universally. Limitations in methods and reporting, however, make it difficult to draw any firm conclusions.

Methods

Randomised controlled trials (RCTs) of the treatment of depression with Chinese herbal medicine were located by searching all of the major Western bibliographic databases. The review located eight trials, three of which were not included in previous reviews. A variety of herbal formulae (combination of herbs) were investigated including Hypericum (St John's wort) and Xia Yao San.

Inclusion criteria:

⇨ A diagnosis of clinical depression using conventional or traditional Chinese criteria

⇨ Interventions using Chinese herbal formulae or single Chinese herbs

⇨ Comparison included placebo, no treatment, or any active treatment

⇨ Improvement in depression (partial or complete alleviation of symptoms).

Exclusion criteria:

⇨ Chinese herbs combined with other complementary therapies

⇨ Participants with depression associated with other conditions.

RCTs were evaluated using two rating scales: the Jadad criteria and the Downs and Black checklist. The effects of the herbal formulae were assessed in seven of the trials by comparing scores on the Hamilton Rating Scale for Depression (HAM-D) before and after treatment. A range of self-report measures and clinical assessment were also used.

Results

It was not possible to combine results to present any meaningful statistics as the herbal formulae and control treatments used, trial duration, and trial design all differed to such an extent. Where changes in depression scores were measured, clinically significant reductions were reported within groups with active treatment – either Chinese herbs or antidepressants and between-group comparisons suggested that Chinese herbs:

⇨ Were more effective than antidepressants – particularly Xiao Yao San and its modifications

⇨ Were comparable to antidepressants

⇨ Did not increase effectiveness but reduced adverse effects or relapse rates when used as an additional therapy with antidepressants

⇨ Were more effective than placebo.

Limitations

There were some major limitations in this review. In the majority of trials the methodological quality was poor and all of the trials were either at risk of bias or the overall risk of bias was unclear:

⇨ It is unclear if the patients selected were representative of the population, as the recruitment process was not reported

⇨ Few, if any, studies provided information on whether intervention and control groups were well matched at baseline, which statistical tests were used and whether participants took the herbal formulae as required

⇨ All studies were described as randomised, but several did not describe how randomisation had been carried out

⇨ Blinding was not always possible and this may have introduced some bias on self-report measures.

There are also problems interpreting the results of these trials:

⇨ Despite herbal formulae having a similar name, they often contain different herbs

⇨ In trials comparing Chinese herbs against antidepressants, it is unclear whether the benefits are a true difference as there was no power calculation

⇨ Little or no detail was provided on dropout, making it difficult to determine the extent to which the Chinese herbs caused reductions in depression

- The longest duration in these trials was 12 weeks, making it impossible to establish long-term efficacy
- All research to date has been conducted in China so it is difficult to translate the results into a Western healthcare context.

Conclusion

Positive results were reported in all of the trials identified and in all but one of the systematic reviews, but despite promising results, particularly for Xia Yao San and its modifications, the effectiveness of Chinese herbal medicine in depression could not be fully substantiated based on current evidence.

The extent to which the results of the study can be used to determine whether Chinese herbs caused reductions in depression (internal validity) or can be generalised to other groups (external validity) is severely limited due to a lack of detail in the research studies. Further well-designed trials would be of interest!

Link

Butler L, Pilkington K. Chinese Herbal Medicine and Depression. Evidence-Based Complementary and Alternative Medicine Volume 2013, Article ID 739716, 14 pages.

Linde K, Berner MM, Kriston L. St John's wort for major depression. Cochrane Database of Systematic Reviews 2008, Issue 4. Art. No.: CD000448. DOI: 10.1002/14651858.CD000448. pub3.

7 May 2013

- The above information is reprinted with kind permission from Dr Jessamy Hibberd. Please visit www.drjessamy. com for further information.

© Dr Jessamy Hibberd 2014

What is traditional acupuncture?

Traditional acupuncture is a healthcare system based on ancient principles which go back nearly two thousand years. It has a very positive model of good health and function, and looks at pain and illness as signs that the body is out of balance. The overall aim of acupuncture treatment, then, is to restore the body's equilibrium. What makes this system so uniquely suited to modern life is that physical, emotional and mental are seen as interdependent, and reflect what many people perceive as the connection between the different aspects of their lives.

Based on traditional belief, acupuncturists are trained to use subtle diagnostic techniques that have been developed and refined for centuries. The focus is on the individual, not their illness, and all the symptoms are seen in relation to each other. Each patient is unique; two people with the same western diagnosis may well receive different acupuncture treatments.

Traditional acupuncturists believe that the underlying principle of treatment is that illness and pain occur when the body's qi, or vital energy, cannot flow freely. There can be many reasons for this; emotional and physical stress, poor nutrition, infection or injury are among the most common. By inserting ultra-fine sterile needles into specific acupuncture points, a traditional acupuncturist seeks to re-establish the free flow of qi to restore balance and trigger the body's natural healing response.

Until the 1940s, when the Chinese Government commissioned the development of a uniform system of diagnosis and treatment, somewhat misleadingly referred to as TCM (Traditional Chinese Medicine), nearly all training had been apprentice-style with masters and within families. The same applied when acupuncture travelled overseas to Japan and South East Asia.

As a consequence of this there are many different styles of acupuncture which share a common root but are distinct and different in their emphasis. You may read of TCM, Five Elements, Stems and Branches, Japanese Meridian Therapy, and many others, all of which have their passionate devotees. The BAcC, though, has long embraced this plurality under the heading 'unity in diversity' and sees the variety of approaches as the mark of a healthy profession.

Traditional acupuncture has a long history of adapting to new cultures in which it is practised. Its growing popularity and acceptance in the West may well promote yet more new and exciting variations on the ancient themes.

A growing body of evidence-based clinical research shows that traditional acupuncture safely treats a wide range of common health problems.

- The above information is reprinted with kind permission from the British Acupuncture Council. Please visit www.acupuncture. org.uk for further information.

© British Acupuncture Council 2014

Ten plants and foods that are natural remedies for illness

By Rachel Moss

If you're concerned about the amount of tablets you take, it might be time to consider using natural remedies.

Natural remedies are alternatives to medicine – they include a variety of therapeutic or preventive health care practices that are thought to help a range of illnesses and improve a person's overall health.

For the answer to your ailment, look no further than your kitchen – many everyday foods are thought to work as natural remedies, either operating as painkillers or even stopping you from getting ill in the first place by boosting your immune system.

With reports claiming that some everyday medicine – such as ibuprofen – can have a serious detrimental effect on your long-term health, we're not surprised that many people are looking for an alternative.

Among other things, studies have shown that natural remedies could help to protect against heart disease, prevent the common cold and help those suffering from arthritis.

Kitchen cupboard natural remedies range from grapes to salmon to ginger.

Garlic is thought to be a superfood in the natural remedy world – studies have shown the stinky herb can aid your respiratory and circulatory system in an unbelievable amount of ways: it could help with high blood pressure, high cholesterol, coronary heart disease, artery hardening and many, many more conditions.

Not only could these natural remedies do your health wonders, they can also improve your diet. And when added to food these products taste great too.

Check out the top natural remedies below but if in doubt, always consult your GP:

Aloe vera

Aloe vera, commonly found as a potted plant in households, produces a gel used to treat skin ailments, such as mild burns, rashes and leg ulcers.

The plant contains acemannan and aloin, which some researchers suspect could be helpful in treating cancer, TLC reports.

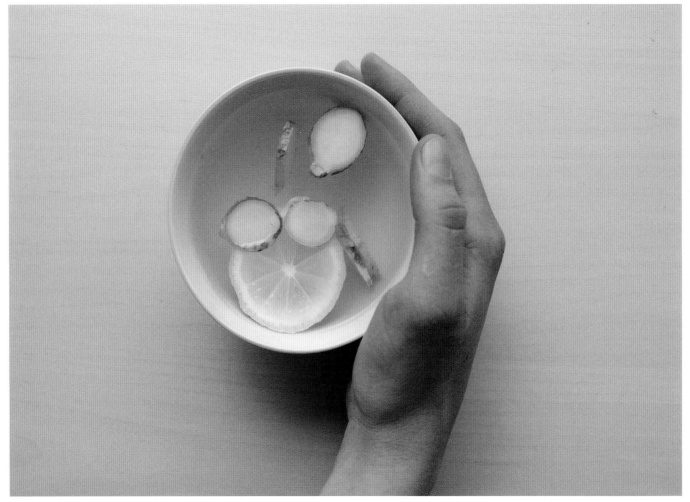

How to use: clean skin or wound thoroughly, break a branch off the plant, apply the juice inside to the skin and cover with a bandage.

Honey

It's not just for Winnie the Pooh any more – unless he has bad skin, that is. A natural antibacterial, honey fights acne while helping skin retain moisture.

How to use: Mix equal parts honey and yogurt to make a face mask, or apply it directly to blemishes.

Ginger

Fresh ginger taken daily has been linked to increased circulation and reduced arthritis pain, *Best Health* says.

Ginger comes in powder and capsule form, and can also be ingested as a tea or as a cooking ingredient. However, ginger can also act as a blood thinner, MSNBC reports, and excessive consumption can lead to adverse side effects, such as an upset stomach.

How to use: In tea, add one teaspoon of grated ginger to boiling water. You can also slice it and add it to meals.

Do not exceed 4 g daily, or 1 g during pregnancy, the University of Maryland Medical Center advises.

Turmeric

'The therapeutic advantages of turmeric and curcumin (its main active component) are almost too numerous to list,' Andrew Weil, M.D. writes in The Huffington Post.

It can aid digestion, has been found to protect the liver and stomach lining, may prevent heart disease and doctors have suggested the spice has the potential to kill cancer cells.

How to use: The daily recommended dose for adults ranges from 1.5 to 3 g of cut root, or 1 to 3 g per day of powdered root, the University of Maryland Medical Center says.

Cranberries

Cranberries (and blueberries, for that matter) contain antioxidants that some believe may prevent urinary tract infections, Charles Patrick Davis, M.D. wrote on MedicineNet.com.

Doctors still prefer to combat UTIs with a more effective low-dose antibiotic, however a daily antibiotic dose generally leads to a higher resistance over time, CNN says.

How to use: The recommended dose is a 300 to 400 mg tablet twice a day, or roughly 240 ml of unsweetened cranberry juice, according to the American Academy of Family Physicians.

Salmon

Studies have found that oily fish has a lot of different health benefits.

Salmon in particular is rich in heart-healthy omega-3 fatty acids – these same compounds may also help reduce pain-promoting inflammation making it a great painkiller alternative for people who suffer with conditions such as rheumatoid arthritis, who have greater risk of heart trouble than people without RA.

Grapes

Research from Ohio University shows that 1 cup of grapes eaten daily can bring relief from backache.

The experts found that grapes contain nutrients that increase blood circulation to the lower back, which in turn alleviates pain.

The humble grape is also high in antioxidants, which are important for eye health and high in water content, which is good for hydration.

High water-content fruits and vegetables are nutrient dense, meaning they provide a large amount of essential nutrients while containing few calories.

Pineapple

If you're using painkillers to deal with menstrual cramps, ditch the tablets and buy some pineapple.

The bromelain in pineapple is known to ease bloated tummy and heaviness. It also improves circulation, stopping cramps and inhibiting inflammation.

It may also help rid the body of inflammatory compounds that contribute to arthritis.

On top of that pineapple can help you give you strong bones, healthy gums and prevent you from getting a cold.

Garlic

Garlic is thought to have many health benefits which range from warding off a cold to protecting your heart against damage.

In the ancient world, garlic played a starring role as painkiller and some still recommend applying it to achey joints.

Studies have shown the food's antioxidants to aid your respiratory and circulatory system in several different ways: it could help with high blood pressure, high cholesterol, coronary heart disease and artery hardening.

23 May 2014

⇨ The above information is reprinted with kind permission from The Huffington Post UK. Please visit www.huffingtonpost.co.uk for further information.

'I feel empowered, in control of my body': four women on fighting cancer with alternative therapies

Four women who have embraced natural therapies in their fight against cancer talk to Anna Moore about their experiences.

Cancer is on the rise. According to a recent report by Macmillan Cancer Support, nearly half of all Britons will receive a diagnosis during their lifetime. Billions of pounds are spent researching and trialling conventional medical treatments, and health advances are made year on year, extending the lives of patients beyond what was previously thought possible.

There is not, however, and probably never will be, a 'golden bullet' – a cure-all for the array of cancers that threaten us. Cancer is a vast and ever-changing problem, and we must keep finding new ways to confront it. We will rightly continue to turn to the medical profession first.

But there is a growing number of people in Britain seeking alternative approaches too, and making their voices heard. It's a controversial area polarising opinion.

According to the breast-cancer charity The Haven, 89 per cent of its service users found that non-medical, complementary therapies (including herbal medicine and nutritional, energy, touch and mind-body therapies) were 'essential' to their recovery.

Sheila Dillon, the presenter of Radio 4's Food Programme and a cancer sufferer, has recently spoken out against the NHS's refusal to accept that diet matters in the fight against cancer.

Kate James, who has worked as an accident and emergency doctor and now runs an integrative medical practice in Northumberland, agrees that diet is important. When her mother and 13-month-old daughter were diagnosed with cancer, she sought ways to complement their conventional chemo- and radiotherapy with alternative treatments.

'I started with diet,' she says, 'taking things out that tend to be difficult to digest and put extra strain on the body and adding in raw food, more juices, chlorophyll-rich foods.' Facing a choice between unproven alternative treatments and imperfect conventional medicine, she chose both.

However, Martin Ledwick, the head information nurse at Cancer Research UK, while able to understand the appeal of alternative treatments, urges caution.

'Alternative cures have always been with us, but the Internet has given them a different channel through which they have gone global,' he says.

'When people set up their blogs or comment in forums about how they've saved themselves, it's very compelling, it may seem convincing, and many people may want to believe it – but it's impossible to know the truth behind it. That person may well have had conventional treatment as well; or the cancer may still be there. Very often, they are trying to sell some magic book, some secret formula – they're making money from it and that's really immoral. Be very careful about what you believe.'

Here four women who turned to natural therapies in their fight against cancer talk about their experiences.

Polly Noble

Polly Noble, 31, lives in Cambridge and has shared her fight against cancer at pollynoble.com.

'I was diagnosed with cervical cancer when I was 24. I had a 3 cm tumour on my cervix and the cancer had spread to my lymph nodes. Surgery, chemotherapy and radiotherapy were the only options I was aware of – and I had them.

'That year was spent asleep or with my head down the loo, but as I got stronger, I started reading about nutrition and alternative therapies and began to think about disease as "dis" "ease", the manifestation of something unresolved, something you created and can cure yourself. As I became more inspired, I began meditation, visualisation, juicing, yoga, coffee enemas. I trained as a life coach and really found my niche.

'In February 2010 doctors found a growth in my neck: the cancer had come back. I was offered radiotherapy, but I said, "Give me six weeks to figure what I'm going to do." I decided against conventional treatment. I wasn't scared; I believed I could heal myself. I went 100-per-cent raw, upped my juicing regime and carried on with visualisation. Within two or three weeks I experienced amazing feelings. I was waking at 5.30am, raring to go.

'For two years I felt great, but then the tumour started growing out of my neck and doctors found secondary cancer in my lungs. I was struggling to swallow, eat or breathe, and by August 2012 my consultant said I might not live to see Christmas. I didn't want chemotherapy – I believe it's a poison and it doesn't deal with the root cause of cancer. I was worried I'd be judged if I went back to conventional medicine. But I do what I can to keep myself alive.

'If I died because I was too stubborn or proud to do something I'd said I wasn't going to do, then more fool me. Right now I'm using a two-pronged attack. I've had chemo to reduce the cancer and alternative therapies to get me through with virtually no side effects. It doesn't have to be one way or the other. You can have the best of alternative and conventional medicine.'

Alyssa Burns-Hill

'When I was diagnosed with breast cancer, my risk factors were practically zero: I was 38, vegetarian, I exercised, I'd had my children young. I had the lump removed and the doctors diagnosed invasive carcinoma, stage one. The hospital recommended radiotherapy and chemotherapy. When asked what I could do to aid my recovery, such as change my diet, they said, 'Nothing' – leave it to the professionals.

'Did I want my path through cancer to be passive or something I was actively involved with, where everything I did was focused on health? I didn't want to give my body chemicals and poisons. My body had created this problem, so if I gave it good things, de-stressed, detoxed, then I felt that I should be able to undo it.

'When I rang the radiotherapy department to cancel my treatments, they were confused. They asked if I'd spoken to my doctor and told me they would have to inform him. My husband and daughters trusted my judgement – but the rest of my family found it difficult to understand and thought I was crazy.

'I call what I did a 21st-century version of Gerson therapy. I had four juices a day, 120 supplements, homeopathic injections and four coffee enemas. I also did yoga, meditation, reiki – a holistic approach. It's not an easy option. The treatment is a full-on, full-time job, and there's no room for anything else.

'After six months I started cutting down the coffee enemas and the number of juices. Now I eat healthily, maintain a high nutritional-supplement intake and love my job as a health specialist. I don't go for check-ups or scans as I don't want the stress. It has been 12 years now.

'I probably feel younger in my 50th year than I did at 38. People say to me, "You're so brave," but it's not about courage or being clever. Going through cancer is about doing what's right for you.'

Hannah Bradley

'I was a salesperson when I was diagnosed with cancer. I ate on the run. I smoked. I had no real symptoms or warning signs. One night in February 2011 I had a grand seizure while I was asleep: arms up in the air, body shaking. My partner, Pete, called an ambulance, and I was rushed to hospital, unconscious. Eventually a CT scan showed a brain tumour, which turned out to be very aggressive, anaplastic astrocytoma.

'I have no memories of that time, from the night of the seizure to coming around from the eight-hour operation to remove the tumour two months later. Looking back now, I was quite naive. I thought that once the surgery was over, the tumour would be gone.

'Then I needed six weeks of radiotherapy, so I did that, thinking this would make me better. It was gruelling – my hair fell out, I had quite a few seizures – then, at the end, a scan showed I still had the remnants of this very aggressive tumour. The life expectancy for people with tumours like this was 18 months.

'All this time, without me knowing, Pete had been looking into things, searching, talking to anyone and everyone who could possibly help. One name kept cropping up: Dr Burzynski.

'At his clinic in Houston he has developed a treatment using anti-cancer compounds he discovered and now manufactures – and is treating aggressive tumours, especially ones in the brain. He's controversial. The medical community claims his work is unscientific and unproven.

'My oncologist didn't want me to go – he wanted to monitor the tumour and maybe give me more radiotherapy in the future. But that was like containing it, not getting rid of it, and the treatment hadn't worked so far. Dr Burzynski seemed to be my only hope of getting rid of the cancer for good.

'The treatment wasn't cheap (about £200,000). Of course we didn't know 100 per cent whether it would work, but I had to believe in something; I wanted to be positive. Pete launched a campaign – friends and family gathered around, held events, our local radio station supported us – and in two months we already had £100,000, enough to start treatment. I'm still so thankful for all that support.

'In December 2011 I flew with Pete to the Burzynski Clinic. The medication is administered directly into your body through a Hickman line 24 hours a day. We were there for seven weeks, and scans showed that in that time the tumour had reduced by 11 per cent. I was absolutely overjoyed.

'Pete and I learnt how to prepare and administer the treatment ourselves and it carried on in Britain for another 18 months. It's not an easy option. My blood was checked twice a week, and I was scanned every six weeks at a private hospital. Most importantly, it seemed to be working. The tumour kept getting smaller, and in January this year it was all gone. I'm now off the treatment but still being monitored.

'Dr Burzynski isn't a miracle worker. There are well-publicised cases of families raising money for children to be treated at the clinic but the children still tragically dying. People have posted on our website that it doesn't work, but I'm convinced that, if we hadn't found him, I wouldn't be here today.

'I wouldn't turn my back on conventional medicine, but I would advise anyone in a situation like mine to look into other options – there could always be another way. If this whole thing has taught me anything, it's that.' A cookbook by Hannah is available at teamhannah.com.

Sarah Shotton

'After all that's happened, I still feel the first diagnosis was the worst. I was 44 and thought the small lump in my breast was a cyst. When we were told it was cancer, I was absolutely devastated. I remember looking at Martin's face – he was white as a sheet – and thinking, "How am I going to tell the kids?" I couldn't see my life past that moment.

'The cancer was HER2-positive, which is less common and tends to be more aggressive. I had three lots of surgery, starting with a lumpectomy, but each time the remaining area wasn't free of cancer, so I finally had a mastectomy.

'Six months of chemo and five weeks of radiotherapy followed. The chemo was horrendous. When it all finished, I went back to "normality" but started to make a few changes. A very close friend who had had breast cancer put me on to Louise Hay, the author of *You Can Heal Your Life*.

'I read *The Secret* by Rhonda Byrne, about the power of positive thinking. I realised I'd lived life on my nerves at 100 mph. I was constantly stressed, drank copious amounts of Diet Coke and coffee. I lived on cake, crisps, ready meals! I started to alter my diet, to give things up and do more things for me.

'Then, in September 2012, a mass I'd noticed in my pelvis – which we first thought was an ovarian cyst – turned out to be a rare cancer: clear cell carcinoma, another primary site, unconnected to the first cancer. Apparently I was just "unfortunate".

'When I had a CT scan, doctors found two liver tumours – secondary cancers from the original breast cancer. The life expectancy isn't good at all, and I was terrified of having chemo again, of putting my body through hell. I thought I'd have to refuse. My lovely friend who'd had breast cancer had now died; she'd taken every drug they'd offered and her suffering had been horrendous.

'With my first diagnosis, I'd put all my faith in the doctors. This time I had the inner strength to question. Instead of letting them choose my path, I wanted to choose it myself. I then heard about Kate James, who runs an integrative practice and can build up your immunity and support you through chemo.

'She met me and made up special prescriptions of medicinal mushrooms, Chinese medicine, herbs – and at the same time I switched to the Hippocrates raw-food diet. I meditate every morning and have weekly acupuncture with a Chinese acupuncturist. By January I felt strong enough to start chemo, and it has been completely different this time. I go into the hospital every week with my green juices, seeds, nuts and lemon water!

'I've had no side effects and feel fantastic, full of energy. Before each session they check my blood counts and liver and kidney functions. The tumours are shrinking: they've gone down by 11 mm. Kate's treatment isn't cheap – about £100 a week.

'My life-insurance policy is the only reason we can afford it, but to me it's essential. I'm now at the stage where I want to stop the chemo, carry on with my diet and alternative treatments and just be monitored by my oncologist. He wants to keep me on the chemo indefinitely, my husband is absolutely terrified, and my sister used to be a pharmacist, so there are intense discussions going on, but I feel empowered, in control of my body.

'If it doesn't work, then it wasn't meant to be – but I need to take the path I believe in.'

20 October 2013

⇨ The above information is reprinted with kind permission from *The Telegraph*. Please visit www.telegraph.co.uk for further information.

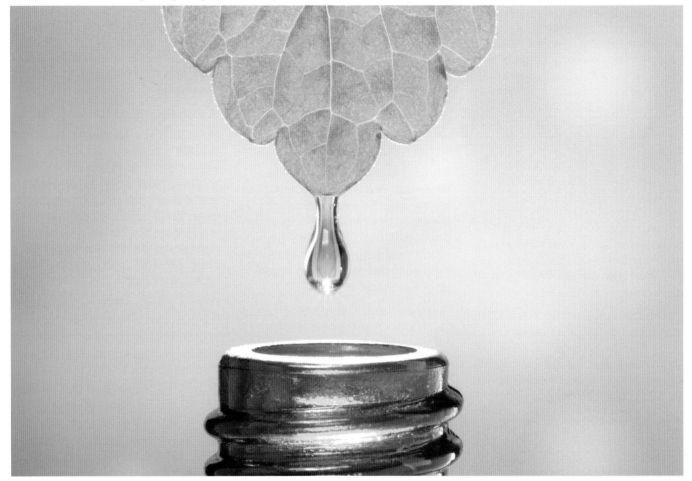

Complementary medicines may put cancer patients' lives at risk

By Nial Wheate Senior Lecturer in Pharmaceutical Chemistry at University of Sydney

Recent German research found that more than 70% of people with cancer supplement their regular hospital treatment with complementary and alternative medicine. More worryingly, many do so without advising their doctor.

This is important because interactions of the complementary medicines and their regular drugs could make cancer treatment ineffective, or worse still, cause toxic side-effects that could lead to death.

The study found a high degree of complementary medicine use by people with cancer across all age groups, and higher use among women than men. A small percentage (8%) of cancer patients were found to only use complementary medicines and shun conventional treatment.

A separate study also found that many parents of children with cancer (30%) also reported giving complementary medicines to their kids.

Studies in the United States, and across other European countries, found similarly high rates of complementary medicine use among cancer patients. Research of this sort hasn't been conducted in Australia, but high complementary medicine use means it's likely the same happens here.

Why people do it

According to the German study, people supplementing their treatment with complementary medicines do so in a variety of ways, and with different products. By far the most popular options are vitamins, metals such as selenium and other trace elements.

Some patients also try non-chemical or drug-based therapies, including prayer, relaxation and physical activity; but these tend to be the least used types of complementary therapies.

More than 50% of the participants in the German study expressed an interest in also using acupuncture or medical herbs, and a quarter were interested in trying mistletoe and homeopathy treatments.

When asked why they were interested in complementary medicines, most people couldn't give a reason, or said they'd used them before being diagnosed with cancer and merely continued that use. Some believed complementary therapies boosted their immune system and helped to 'detoxify' their body.

Interestingly, more than a third of the German patients reported using complementary therapies simply because it enabled them to do something for themselves; it let them feel more in control of their treatment.

There's considerable debate about the usefulness of complementary therapies, but what is more worrying about all three studies into complementary therapy use is that it happens without the knowledge of the patient's doctor.

When asked about the source of their information on complementary medicines, the four most common responses in the German study were television and radio, family and friends, books, and the Internet.

The three least used sources of information were, in decreasing order, doctors, non-medical practitioners and pharmacists. In total, fewer than 10% of the people in the study using complementary medicines stated they gained information on them from health professionals.

This could be a problem because there's no guarantee that popular sources of information about complementary therapies are accurate. Australian research from 2008 found that much of the information available in the media about complementary therapies is either incomplete or inaccurate.

Lurking dangers

Combining complementary medicine with conventional cancer treatment opens up the possibility of drug interactions that can make cancer treatment ineffective. Worse still, the drugs may interact to exacerbate side-effects of chemotherapy, which can be so severe they endanger the person's life.

What's more, many complementary medicines, particularly those marketed herbal or all-natural, can contain ingredients not listed on the labels. So people don't know what they are taking.

The Therapeutic Goods Administration regularly bans and issues safety advisories for complementary medicine products that patients are buying over the Internet because they contain unlisted, often prescription-only, ingredients.

Cancer patients should discuss any medicines they plan to use that are outside their normal treatment plan with their doctor. Many complementary medicines they choose will be safe.

Regardless of efficacy, complementary medicines provide people with an important way to gain a feeling of ownership over their treatment. Doctors will always be supportive of their patients and can help choose complementary medicines that are effective and safe for them to use.

8 September 2013

⇨ The above information is reprinted with kind permission from The Conversation. Please visit www.theconversation.com for further information.

What does the public really think about homeopathy?

There is nothing more likely to raise the hackles of any self-respecting rationalist than to be confronted with the latest celebrity story about the miraculous healing power of homeopathy or some other 'alternative' or 'complementary' quackery. Or, embarrassingly, to discover that some of your best friends are also devotees.

This isn't a new bugbear in response to some kind of New Age, middle-class hippiedom. Charles Darwin wrote in a letter to a cousin:

You speak about Homeopathy; which is a subject which makes me more wrath, even than does Clairvoyance: clairvoyance so transcends belief, that one's ordinary faculties are put out of question, but in Homeopathy common sense and common observation come into play, & both these must go to the Dogs, if the infinitesimal doses have any effect whatever.

There is no serious scientific debate about the efficacy of homeopathy.

It performs no better than placebo and is based on principles wholly at odds with established scientific understanding. Nevertheless, it whips up what might seem like a disproportionate amount of political controversy.

Health Secretary Jeremy Hunt (yes, the man in charge of UK national health policy) is a known sympathiser and got into hot water for allowing Prince Charles to lobby him about prescribing it on the NHS.

A newly appointed public health shadow minister, Luciana Berger, was 'forced to renounce' previously positive views.

And earlier in 2013, Chief Scientist Mark Walport called homeopathy 'nonsense', while his predecessor, John Beddington, said that NHS spending on homeopathy was the only issue where ministers had 'fundamentally ignored' his scientific advice. Sally Davis, England's Chief Medical Officer, said that the taxpayers' £4 million

would be better spent on proven treatments as hospitals suffer painful cutbacks.

Our survey says

Yet while binary opposition between support for homeopathy (and other complementary and alternative medicine (CAM) treatments) is how public debate is framed, it is far from clear that the public thinks and does the same.

In research we carried out using the Wellcome Monitor Survey, we interviewed a random sample of 1,179 UK adults aged over 18 about homeopathy and other CAMs. We also wanted to know why some people chose or not to use these treatments.

A slim majority of the group reported that they had never used CAM. The most popular treatments with the remaining half were herbal medicines, homeopathy and acupuncture.

A quarter of the respondents who reported that they had never used homeopathy said this was because they hadn't heard of it; a third because they had never been advised to take the treatment and/or that they'd never had an illness that required it; and 3% said it was because homeopathic remedies were too expensive.

Less than a quarter of non-users said that they had avoided homeopathy because they didn't believe that it worked, or that conventional medicine worked better.

Of course, this may be in part a result of asking a question in a survey of this kind: it is quite hard for people to single out reasons for not doing things.

The most telling statistics emerged when we asked people that said they had used homeopathy why they had: 49% said they were 'willing to try anything and didn't think it could

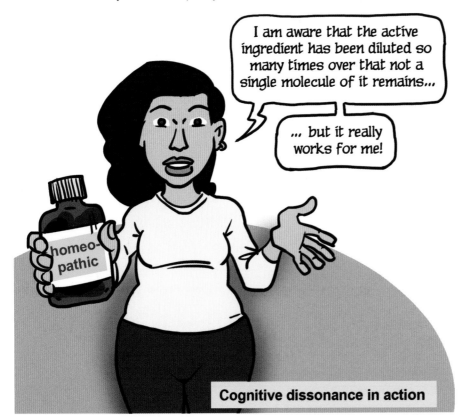

I am aware that the active ingredient has been diluted so many times over that not a single molecule of it remains...

... but it really works for me!

homeo-pathic

Cognitive dissonance in action

do any harm'. Only 16% said it was because they believed they worked better than conventional medicine. This means that only around 3% of the population have used homeopathy from a belief that it works where conventional medicine doesn't. The rest either have not used it, or used it for other reasons.

Disaffected, conventional and dissonant

To explore this further, we used a statistical modelling technique called latent class analysis, which helps identify groups of persons that are similar to each other in their profile of survey responses. We selected questions for analysis based on the key dimensions of public debate: the importance of science education, belief in the effectiveness of homeopathy, use of CAM, trust in medical doctors and optimism about medical advances in general.

We found that we could split the public into three groups. The first, who we called the 'disaffected', comprise just under 30%.

They are generally pessimistic about medicine, don't see the value of science education and don't believe in the efficacy of homeopathy either.

A second 'conventional' group, accounting for just over 30% of citizens, are likely to be supportive and trusting of conventional medicine, reject CAM and value science education.

The third and largest group (just over 40% of the population) is the most interesting. This group is likely to have used CAM and to think that homeopathy is effective. Yet they are overwhelmingly trusting of medical doctors, value science education and are optimistic about medical advances. We call this group the 'dissonants' (although they are unlikely to call themselves that).

So what makes it likely that someone will be a dissonant rather than a conventional? Women are more likely to be found in the dissonant group. Interestingly, people who are better educated

are also more likely to be found in this group (although from a set of questions we posed in the survey, those with a science qualification and who did better in a scientific quiz are less likely to be included), along with those that think that there's too little regulation of medical research.

At odds in the public mind?

Our research suggests that nearly half of the public don't believe and act as if CAM and conventional medicine are at odds. Coupled with the significant global industry that has grown up around CAM, it is easy to see why politicians have been unwilling to respond to the clear evidence that homeopathy and CAM are ineffective. In the US, it's a $34 billion industry where half of people report using them.

The competition between proponents and opponents of CAM in all likelihood is set to continue. But there's some evidence that better science education can help people to distinguish between scientific and pseudo-scientific claims, and it appears that at least some of the openness to CAM might stem from concerns about how medical research is regulated. And it is these that might hold the key to who ultimately comes out of the ring in better shape.

The research on which this article is based was carried out with Paul Stoneman, Patrick Sturgis and Elissa Sibley.

13 January 2014

⇨ The above information is reprinted with kind permission from The Conversation. Please visit www.theconversation.com for further information.

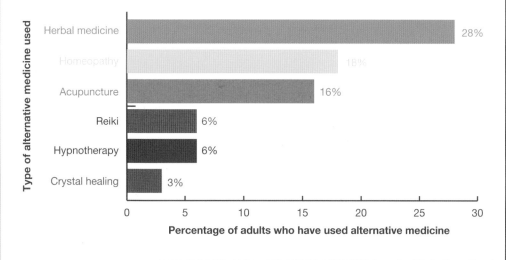

Adults' experience of using alternative medicines

Had used any

Not used any

= 5 %

Type of alternative medicine ever used by respondents who had used any

Type of alternative medicine used

Herbal medicine	28%
Homeopathy	18%
Acupuncture	16%
Reiki	6%
Hypnotherapy	6%
Crystal healing	3%

Percentage of adults who have used alternative medicine

Source: Butt S, Clery E, Abeywardana V, Phillips M (2009) Wellcome Trust Monitor Survey Report. National Centre for Social Research (Updated November 2012).

Homeopathy on the NHS is 'mad' says outgoing scientific adviser

The use of homeopathy by the NHS has been described as 'mad' by a former government scientific adviser who retired from his post last week.

By Richard Gray, Science Correspondent

Professor Sir John Beddington criticised the Government for ignoring his advice against the use of homeopathic remedies by GPs and NHS-run hospitals.

Sir John, who retired as chief scientific adviser to the Government on 1 April, expressed frustration that ministers had continued to allow taxpayers, money to be used to fund such treatments despite them having 'no scientific basis'.

Homeopathy, which uses highly diluted extracts from plants, herbs and minerals to treat diseases, costs the NHS between £4 million and £12 million a year.

The Prince of Wales is among the advocates of homeopathy while Jeremy Hunt, the health secretary is also known to be a supporter, but it has been widely debunked by the medical community.

Sir John said the provision of homeopathic remedies on the NHS was the only occasion during his five years as chief scientific adviser that his views had been 'fundamentally ignored' by the Government.

He said: 'The only one I could think of was homeopathy, which is mad. It has no underpinning of scientific basis.

'In fact all of the science points to the fact that it is not at all sensible.

'The clear evidence is saying this is wrong, but homeopathy is still used on the NHS.'

Homeopathy is based on the idea that illnesses can be treated by substances that produce similar symptoms.

For example, sleeplessness could be treated by diluted doses of coffee because when drunk in normal amounts it can keep people awake.

In some cases it is claimed to be able to treat serious illnesses including cancer.

The scientific consensus, however, is that homeopathic treatments only work through the placebo effect, where patients experience an improvement in their condition despite not being given any active ingredient or medical treatment.

The British Medical Association has described homeopathy as 'witchcraft' while earlier this year Professor Dame Sally Davies, the chief medical officer, described it as 'rubbish'.

The Parliamentary Science and Technology Committee also concluded in 2010 that the 'Government should stop allowing the funding of homeopathy on the NHS'.

There are currently five homeopathic hospitals run by the NHS in the UK – one each in Bristol, London and Glasgow.

An appointment with a homeopath and a course of homeopathic pills are estimated to cost around £140 per patient.

Although the NHS does not publish how much is spent on homeopathy, it spent £121,000 on homeopathic prescriptions in 2010.

The British Homeopathic Association says £4 million of public money is spent each year, although it has been claimed that the figure could be as much as £12 million a year.

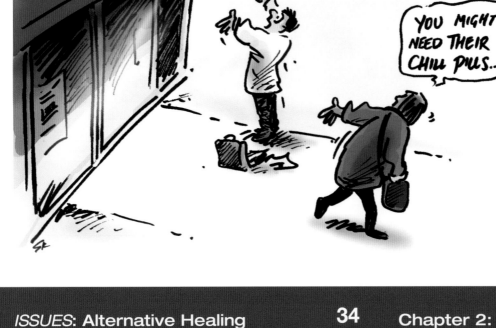

A spokesman for the Department of Health said: 'The Department of Health does not maintain a position on any particular complementary or alternative therapy including homeopathy.

'It is the responsibility of local NHS organisations to make decisions on the commissioning and funding of any healthcare treatments for NHS patients, such as homeopathy.

'This should take account of issues to do with safety, clinical evidence and cost-effectiveness and the availability of suitably qualified and regulated practitioners.'

Dr Sara Eames, president of the Faculty of Homeopathy, insisted that homeopathy gave positive results to patients.

She said: 'Professor Beddington fails to mention that many more randomised clinical trials in homeopathy have produced positive results than negative.

'Instead of dismissing homeopathy, surely it would be far more sensible to carry out research into why doctors and other healthcare professionals trained in homeopathy and working within the NHS, regularly see such positive patient outcomes following homeopathic treatment.'

Sir John, who was talking at the Science Media Centre in London, also warned that in some cases excessive regulations that used a precautionary approach to risk were creating problems.

He said that European rulings that used this approach, such as banning plastic bottles containing the chemical Bisphenol A in 2010 and the more recent attempt to ban pesticides thought to kill honey bees, risked doing more harm than good.

He said the Icelandic volcano eruption that threw ash into the atmosphere and resulted in thousands of flights being cancelled for over a week, was a good example of this.

He said: 'This is the other thing that worries me – and you can see an example in the volcanic ash where the problems were actually caused by regulation.

'The regulations said that if there was ash in the air at any concentration you did not fly. It's crazy. It depends how long you fly through it, what the concentration is.

'There are a whole series of regulations affecting us and we need to be thinking about it.

'There is a real danger of what is happening in the EU in general is an over use of the precautionary principle.

'The banning of Bisphenol A in baby bottles is another example of this. To be frank, the only way you can harm babies with Bisphenol A bottles is to beat them over the head with them.

'With the bans on agrochemicals, they are taking a hazard-based approach and introducing regulations that say stop using them. I think this is the over use and illegitimate use of the precautionary principle.

'It is a fine line and needs some debate.'

9 April 2013

⇨ The above information is reprinted with kind permission from *The Telegraph*. Please visit www. telegraph.co.uk for further information.

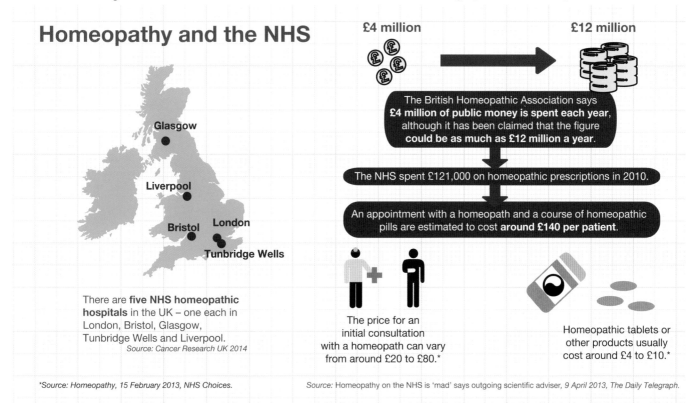

Homeopathy and the NHS

Glasgow

Liverpool

Bristol   London

Tunbridge Wells

There are **five NHS homeopathic hospitals** in the UK – one each in London, Bristol, Glasgow, Tunbridge Wells and Liverpool.
Source: Cancer Research UK 2014

£4 million   £12 million

The British Homeopathic Association says **£4 million of public money is spent each year**, although it has been claimed that the figure **could be as much as £12 million a year**.

The NHS spent £121,000 on homeopathic prescriptions in 2010.

An appointment with a homeopath and a course of homeopathic pills are estimated to cost **around £140 per patient**.

The price for an initial consultation with a homeopath can vary from around £20 to £80.*

Homeopathic tablets or other products usually cost around £4 to £10.*

*Source: Homeopathy, 15 February 2013, NHS Choices.

Source: Homeopathy on the NHS is 'mad' says outgoing scientific adviser, *9 April 2013, The Daily Telegraph.*

He's at it again: Prince Charles accused of lobbying Health Secretary over homeopathy

Prince Charles has apparently been lobbying Jeremy Hunt about the controversial alternative treatment, much to the annoyance of Labour MPs.

Prince Charles was last night urged to stay out of the debate over homeopathy on the NHS, amid claims that he had lobbied the Health Secretary in favour of the controversial alternative treatment.

Labour MPs reacted with fury at the revelation that the heir to the throne had met Jeremy Hunt last week, with NHS support for homeopathy believed to be on the agenda. The disclosure of the Prince's latest communications with senior politicians came days after judges ruled that the public has no right to know the contents of 27 letters he had written to ministers over several years, in an attempt to influence policy decisions.

Prince Charles is a long-term advocate of homeopathy, which involves treating patients with highly diluted substances 'with the aim of triggering the body's natural system of healing'. Mr Hunt once told a constituent that 'it ought to be available [on the NHS] where a doctor and patient believe that a homeopathic treatment may be of benefit'.

'Prince Charles is believed to be frustrated with the Government's failure to force through a register of practitioners of herbal and Chinese medicine'

Earlier this year the Government's new chief scientific adviser, Sir Mark Walport, dismissed homeopathy as 'nonsense', but critics have complained that the NHS is still spending millions of pounds a year on a therapy they claim has no effect on patients.

Despite Mr Hunt's support for homeopathy, Prince Charles is believed to be frustrated with the Government's failure to force through a register of practitioners of herbal and Chinese medicine.

But the Birmingham Labour MP Steve McCabe said it was 'strange' that the heir to the throne should be able to lobby the Health Secretary on such a controversial issue. 'It is even more extraordinary that he should be allowed to do this in secret... I can't see how it isn't in the public interest for the rest of us to know,' he said. His colleague, Paul Flynn, claimed the Prince had a duty to remain neutral, particularly over a hugely controversial issue involving public spending and the health of the nation. 'People are entitled to believe what they want, but having the heir to the throne attempting to influence the spending of precious NHS resources on a service he probably doesn't use at all is ludicrous... Prince Charles should not be interfering; he is in training for his role as monarch and the first lesson is to put a bandage round his mouth and to keep it there at all times,' he said.

'Prince Charles is a long-term advocate of homeopath'

Homeopaths claim they can treat a range of conditions. But a critical report from the Health Select Committee in 2010 raised questions over its effectiveness. It said: 'Homeopathy should not be funded on the NHS.' Governments have since avoided endorsing it, but clinics and trusts are free to offer homeopathic treatments.

The Tory MP David Tredinnick, a supporter of homeopathy who also sits on the Health Select Committee, said he was not concerned about Prince Charles's intervention, as 'he is probably as well placed as anybody in the country to comment on this'. Speaking on the BBC, Mr Tredinnick said: 'We should do what they do in the rest of the world, which is to take [homeopathy] seriously.'

But David Colquhoun, a pharmacologist at University College London, said homeopathy was 'utter nonsense'. 'Homeopathic remedies contain nothing whatsoever. The Americans have spent $2 billion investigating these things... they haven't found a single one that works,' he said.

Clarence House confirmed the Prince had met Mr Hunt last week, but neither they nor the Department of Health would give details of the discussions.

21 July 2013

⇨ The above information is reprinted with kind permission from *The Independent*. Please visit www.independent.co.uk for further information.

The placebo effect

When a person uses any type of health treatment and sees an improvement in their symptoms, they may be experiencing the placebo effect. That's why it's important to be aware of the placebo effect when judging the effectiveness of a treatment, or when using one ourselves.

The placebo effect is about the power of the mind to influence the body.

It can occur when a person uses any kind of health treatment, either conventional or complementary and alternative.

It can affect all of us, whether we know about the placebo effect or not.

It's important to be aware of the placebo effect when choosing complementary and alternative treatments. That is because if we choose a complementary or alternative treatment that does not work – and causes only a placebo effect – we may miss out on more effective treatments.

What is the placebo effect?

For hundreds of years, doctors have known that when a patient with a health condition expects their symptoms to improve, they often do improve.

Today, we know that patients who are given empty injections or pills that they believe contain medicine can experience improvement in a wide range of health conditions. This kind of fake or empty medicine is often called a placebo, and the improvement that results is called the placebo effect.

The placebo effect is an example of how our expectations and beliefs can cause real change in our physical bodies. It's a phenomenon that we don't completely understand. But we can see it working in all kinds of ways, and all kinds of circumstances.

The placebo effect at work

Take one well-known example based on a physical feeling we are all familiar with: pain.

In 1996, scientists assembled a group of students and told them that they were going to take part in a study of a new painkiller, called 'trivaricaine'. Trivaricaine was a brown lotion to be painted on the skin, and smelled like a medicine. But the students were not told that, in fact, trivaricaine contained only water, iodine, and thyme oil, none of which are painkilling medicines. It was a fake – or placebo – painkiller. Read an abstract of the study: *Mechanisms of Placebo Pain Reduction*.

With each student, the trivaricaine was painted on one index finger, and the other left untreated. In turn, each index finger was squeezed in a vice. The students reported significantly less pain in the treated finger, even though trivaricaine was a fake.

In this example, expectation and belief produced real results. The students expected the 'medicine' to kill pain: and, sure enough, they experienced less pain. This is the placebo effect.

Placebo medicine has even been shown to cause stomach ulcers to heal faster than they otherwise would.

These amazing results show that the placebo effect is real, and powerful. They mean that fake or placebo treatments can cause real improvements in health conditions: improvements we can see with our own eyes.

Experiencing the placebo effect is not the same as being 'tricked', or being foolish. The effect can happen to everyone, however intelligent, and whether they know about the placebo effect or not.

CAM and the placebo effect

Evidence about a treatment is gathered by conducting fair tests. In these tests, scientists find out whether a treatment causes an improvement beyond the improvement caused by the placebo effect alone.

Evidence plays an important role in mainstream medicine. This means that when you use many conventional medicines, you can be sure that there is evidence that they work.

When patients experience improvement after using a healthcare treatment that has not been proven to work, they may be experiencing only the placebo effect.

Of course, improvement in a health condition due to the placebo effect is still improvement, and that is always welcome.

But it is important to remember that for many health conditions, there are treatments that work better than placebo treatments. If you choose a treatment that provides only a placebo effect, you will miss out on the benefit that a better treatment would provide.

Check the evidence

The only way to know whether a health treatment works better than a placebo treatment is by checking the evidence.

You can learn more about evidence, how it is gathered, and why it is important in *CAM: what is evidence?* on the NHS website.

You can learn about the evidence for many of the best-known complementary and alternative medicines in the Health A-Z pages on the NHS website.

23 November 2012

⇨ The above information is reprinted with kind permission from NHS Choices. Please visit www.nhs.uk for further information.

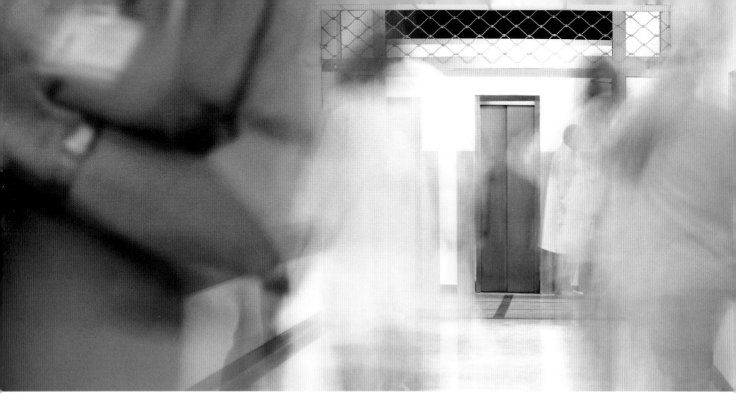

Pregnant women using alternative therapies urged to tell their doctors

Natural 'not always safe', warn experts, as study shows 90% of pregnant Australian women use complementary treatments.

Doctors are urging pregnant Australian women to tell them about their use of complementary and alternative therapies after a new study found 90% are using such treatments, often on the advice of their friends and families.

Using data from the Australian Longitudinal Study on Women's Health pregnancy sub-survey of more than 1,800 women, researchers found almost half consulted a complementary and alternative medicine (CAM) practitioner and almost 90% used a CAM product during pregnancy. More than 40% were influenced to do so by family and friends, while about half were influenced by their own use of CAM in the past.

'It is noteworthy that women were not significantly influenced by professional maternity healthcare providers when deciding to consult a CAM practitioner,' the study said.

Pregnant women experiencing back pain, sciatica, nausea or who were preparing for labour were most likely to take the advice of friends and family to see CAM practitioners, the researchers from Sydney and Queensland found. The findings were published in the *Journal of Alternative and Complementary Medicine*.

Study lead author and research scholar from the University of Technology's Australian Research Centre in Complementary and Integrative Medicine, Jane Frawley, said women were also using the Internet for advice on complementary medicine, but not as much as she anticipated.

'This may be due to issues around trust,' she said.

'Women may not always trust the Internet, but a friend or family member saying that they found a particular remedy helpful for a particular pregnancy symptom is a powerful endorsement.'

Many of the therapies women use are safe or have no effect. But Frawley said women should be aware that natural did not always mean safe, and some were potentially harmful, especially during pregnancy.

She was concerned women may be delaying or avoiding conventional treatment for a potentially dangerous condition, such as a urinary tract infection. Women may be worried about being judged for their CAM use by their GPs, she said, despite many obstetricians and midwives being open-minded towards some complementary treatments.

'Women should always discuss their use of CAM with their maternity healthcare provider,' she said.

President of the Royal Australian College of General Practitioners, Dr Liz Marles, said it was important for doctors to be non-judgemental about use of unconventional treatments.

'Most women are really trying to do the right thing for their baby and doctors need to understand that,' she said. But doctors also needed to be honest if a patient's CAM use could be harmful, she said.

'I would definitely like to know if my pregnant patients were receiving any form of spinal manipulation, or if they were taking any herbal remedies, because they often contain some quite potent substances.'

The Australian Natural Therapies Association, whose members include homeopaths, naturopaths and aromatherapists, state on their website that their members have full access to an interactions database covering more than 700 herb-drug, supplement-drug, and food-drug interactions. They say the website is updated weekly.

Royal Australian and New Zealand College of Obstetricians and Gynaecologists vice-president, associate professor Steve Robson, said he saw CAM use among his patients 'all the time'. Patients often had no idea what they were taking, he said.

'Very recently I had a patient come in with a bottle of something given to her by a CAM practitioner and asked if it was safe to take it, but I had no idea what was in it – it was impossible to tell what was in it,' he said. Another pregnant patient told him she was taking a herbal remedy for a bowel problem, despite much more effective conventional treatments being available.

But many others patients did not disclose their use of alternative therapies at all, he said.

'Doctors prescribe treatments within a strong regulatory framework, where drugs are rated for safety and we know how to use them and of any potential side-effects,' Robson said.

'Women will check with me if it's safe to take a panadol, but won't disclose less evidence-based treatments.'

Some CAM substances, including herbal remedies, could affect the hormones or electrolyte balance of pregnant women, he said. He was particularly concerned about non-health professionals attempting to turn babies from the breech position, rather than performing the potentially fraught procedure in a hospital with doctors and midwives present.

Robson believes women may be influenced by CAM practitioners because they have more time than doctors to sit down and talk to them.

'Doctors and midwives are often rushed, but CAM practitioners will make a big fuss over someone and spend up to an hour with them,' he said.

'That must be very appealing. But pregnancy can be such a time of vulnerability, and some of these alternative treatments have no evidence base whatsoever and have the potential for downsides.'

13 June 2013

⇨ The above information is reprinted with kind permission from *The Guardian.* Please visit www.theguardian.com for further information.

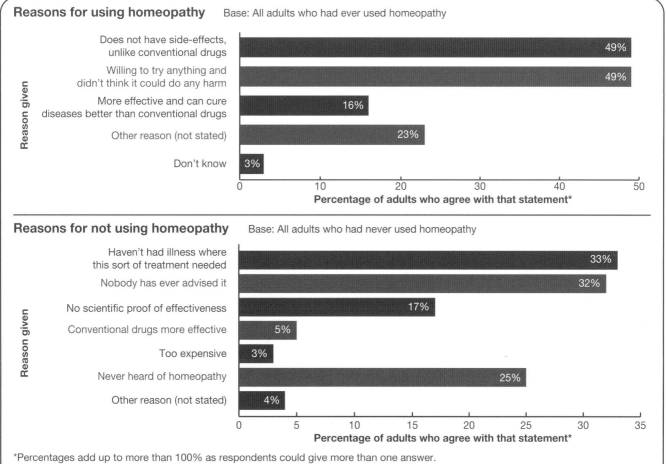

Reasons for using homeopathy   Base: All adults who had ever used homeopathy

Reason given

	Percentage
Does not have side-effects, unlike conventional drugs	49%
Willing to try anything and didn't think it could do any harm	49%
More effective and can cure diseases better than conventional drugs	16%
Other reason (not stated)	23%
Don't know	3%

Percentage of adults who agree with that statement*

Reasons for not using homeopathy   Base: All adults who had never used homeopathy

Reason given

	Percentage
Haven't had illness where this sort of treatment needed	33%
Nobody has ever advised it	32%
No scientific proof of effectiveness	17%
Conventional drugs more effective	5%
Too expensive	3%
Never heard of homeopathy	25%
Other reason (not stated)	4%

Percentage of adults who agree with that statement*

*Percentages add up to more than 100% as respondents could give more than one answer.

Source: Butt S, Clery E, Abeywardana V, Phillips M (2009) Wellcome Trust Monitor Survey Report. National Centre for Social Research (Updated November 2012).

Key facts

- Approximately three million people undergo acupuncture treatment in the UK each year. (page 1)

- Homeopathic medicines are prepared by serial dilution in steps of 1:10 or 1:100, denoted by the Latin numbers x and c, respectively. (page 1)

- The Faculty of Homeopathy regulates the training and practise of homeopathy by medically qualified doctors. There is a published list of doctors who are members of the faculty: The most experienced homeopaths have the qualifications FFHom or MFHom and the qualification LFHom indicates a doctor who may use homeopathy in a limited way for minor ailments. (page 2)

- Acupuncture originated in China, probably more than 4,000 years ago. (page 2)

- A complementary therapy means you can use it alongside your conventional medical treatment... An alternative therapy is generally used instead of conventional medical treatment. (page 6)

- There are more than 150,000 registered medical doctors with additional CAM certification in Europe and more than 180,000 registered and certified non-medical CAM practitioners. (page 10)

- Ten to 20% of the UK population visit a complementary medicine practitioner each year and between £1.5–5 billion per annum is spent on therapies or products allied to complementary medicine. (page 11)

- [As from 1 July 2012,] there are only five appropriately qualified pharmacies under the regulations which can dispense the four dozen or so formally registered potions that can be legally sold. All other homeopathic prescribing and supply not involving a face-to-face consultation with a registered homeopath will be unlawful. (page 12)

- According to new research carried out by TRAFFIC, parts of 1,537 tigers have been seized in illegal trade across 13 tiger range countries in the 14 years between 2000 and 2013. (page 17)

- Private practitioners of complementary therapies can charge up to £60 or more per hour. These costs vary from place to place within the UK – for example, treatments are usually more expensive in cities. (page 19)

- In recent surveys, 85 per cent of medical students, 76 per cent of GPs and 69 per cent of hospital doctors have said they feel that complementary therapies should be made available on the NHS. (page 20)

- Since April 2011, all manufactured herbal medicines have to be registered under a new scheme, known as the Traditional Herbal Registration (THR). (page 21)

- 90% of respondents said that should they be diagnosed with a terminal illness, they would consider complementary therapy to help them to deal with the symptoms. (page 23)

- Aloe vera, commonly found as a potted plant in households, produces a gel used to treat skin ailments, such as mild burns, rashes and leg ulcers. (page 25)

- Recent German research found that more than 70% of people with cancer supplement their regular hospital treatment with complementary and alternative medicine. (page 31)

- [A survey] we asked people that said they had used homeopathy why they had: 49% said they were 'willing to try anything and didn't think it could do any harm'. Only 16% said it was because they believed they worked better than conventional medicine. This means that only around 3% of the population have used homeopathy from a belief that it works where conventional medicine doesn't. The rest either have not used it, or used it for other reasons. (page 33)

- An appointment with a homeopath and a course of homeopathic pills are estimated to cost around £140 per patient. (page 34)

- Although the NHS does not publish how much is spent on homeopathy, it spent £121,000 on homeopathic prescriptions in 2010. (page 34)

- The British Homeopathic Association says £4 million of public money is spent each year, although it has been claimed that the figure could be as much as £12 million a year. (page 34)

- There are five NHS homeopathic hospitals in the UK – one each in London, Bristol, Glasgow, Tunbridge Wells and Liverpool. (page 35)

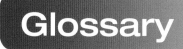

Glossary

10:23 campaign

The 10:23 campaign consists of a group of people who are sceptical about the claims of homeopaths, particularly with regard to the efficacy of their products. In January 2010, members of the group took part in a demonstration outside the Boots chain of chemists, during which they took a massive overdose of Boots-stocked homeopathic remedies in order to show that they had no effect on health. Although the group claimed the protest was a success, the British Homeopathic Association condemned it as 'irresponsible'.

Acupuncture

An ancient practice which involves inserting sterile needles into strategic points on the human body with the aim of relieving pain and other negative symptoms.

Aromatherapy

Aromatherapy utilises scented 'essential oils', which practitioners claim will induce certain moods or promote good health (e.g. calming/relaxation). They can be inhaled, used as a massage oil or occasionally ingested. There are over 400 different essential oils and they are extracted from plants all over the world. Popular oils used include chamomile, lavender, rosemary and tea tree.

British Homeopathic Association

A charity who works closely with the Faculty of Homeopathy to promote and develop the study and practise of homeopathy. Their aim is to advance education and research about homeopathy and to promote patient access to homeopathy (they believe that healthcare systems should have homeopathy available as a treatment option).

Chiropractic

Chiropractors are practitioners of complementary medicine, and are legally-recognised professionals just like doctors and nurses. Chiropractic teaches that spinal disorders can affect the health of the body generally, and seeks to treat these through a combination of methods, including spinal adjustment and manipulation; massage; exercises and lifestyle counselling.

Complementary and Alternative Medicine (CAM)

CAM includes a wide range of therapies and practices that are outside the mainstream of medicine: for example, homeopathy, herbal remedies, acupuncture, reflexology, reiki and traditional Chinese medicine. Complementary medicine uses therapies that work alongside conventional medicine. Alternative medicine includes treatments that are not currently considered part of evidence-based Western medicine. However, as the distinction between the two is not clear-cut, the term complementary and alternative medicine (CAM) is now widely used to include both approaches. The effectiveness of some forms of CAM is often hotly debated.

Holism

A Greek word meaning 'all' or 'whole'. Holistic health teaches that an individual should be considered as a whole and offered medical treatments as such: hence the oft-cited CAM principle that complementary and alternative therapies treats the individual, not the disease. In alternative medicine, a holistic approach will take all of an individual's needs – physical, psychological, spiritual and social – into account when considering the causes of an illness and the best way to treat it.

Homeopathy

A form of alternative medicine in which practitioners use highly diluted substances to treat their patients. The thinking behind this practice is that when substances known to cause certain symptoms are delivered to patients exhibiting those same symptoms in a highly diluted form, the substances will be effective as a treatment. According to the Society of Homeopaths' website, a homeopathic remedy of 30C contains less than one part per million of the original substance. While practitioners and patients are vocal supporters of the benefits of homeopathy, its critics claim that there is a lack of scientific and clinical evidence to support it and that it offers little more than a placebo effect.

Massage therapy

A 'therapeutic touch' which can be used for health benefits, such as helping people relax, making people feel energised, relieving tension or helping ease muscle pain/stiffness. There are many different massage styles and techniques which involve the use of a varying number of movements and pressures on different parts of the body. Some of the most common types of massage are Swedish massage, deep tissue massage and Indian head massage – each have their own specialist techniques that tackle different ailments.

Osteopathy

Osteopaths are practitioners of complementary medicine, and are legally-recognised professionals just like doctors and nurses. Osteopathic principles teach that treating bones, muscles and joints can aid the body in repairing itself.

Placebo

A placebo is a substance administered to patients containing no active ingredients: for example, a sugar pill or saline solution. However, the patient taking the placebo is led to believe that it is a medicine which will have a positive effect on certain symptoms they are displaying. The 'placebo effect' refers to an improvement in symptoms brought about by a patient's belief that the inactive substance they are taking will cure or improve their illness. Critics of certain types of alternative medicine, for example homeopathy, believe that the treatments given to patients by practitioners are little more than placebos.

Yoga

With historical origins in ancient Indian philosophy, yoga aims to transform the mind and body through physical, mental and spiritual disciplines. With regular practise, the exercise of yoga is meant to bring health benefits such as increased energy levels, relief from muscle pain and stiffness and improved circulation.

Assignments

Brainstorming

⇨ In small groups, discuss what you know about alternative medicine. Consider the following points:

- What is complementary and alternative medicine (CAM)?

- What are the various forms of CAM?

- How does CAM differ from conventional medicine?

- What is the placebo effect?

Research

⇨ Using *How to choose a CAM practitioner* (pages 8-9), find a registered CAM practitioners in your area. What kind of treatments do they offer? How much do they cost? Make some notes and compare with your classmates.

⇨ Investigate the use of alternative/traditional medicines and therapies in other countries around the world. How do opinions on alternative and conventional treatments vary from country to country? Write a summary of your findings.

⇨ Find out about the use of complementary therapy in palliative care. How can complementary therapies improve patients' quality of life towards the end of their lives? Make a bullet point list of your findings.

⇨ Homeopathy has been offered on the National Health Service since it was founded in 1948. Research the history of homeopathy on the NHS. Which treatments are recommended? Feedback to your class.

⇨ Take a poll of your class and ask them about their experience of using alternative medicine. Questions you might want to consider asking: what do you really think about homeopathy? Have you used any alternative medicines? If yes, what type of alternative medicine have you used? If no, why not? Using the data you have collected, create graphs and write up a report with your findings.

Design

⇨ Draw a diagram of the human body and identify which complementary therapies are used to treat different parts.

⇨ Imagine you are starting a new practice that specialises in alternative therapies. Think of a name for your practice, give yourself a logo and create some posters to promote your new business.

⇨ Design a leaflet that shows which natural remedies can be used to help treat certain ailments. Read *Ten plants and foods that are natural remedies for illness* (pages 26-27) for ideas.

⇨ Design an informative poster which highlights the special laws surrounding CAM and how the practice is regulated.

⇨ Choose an article from this book and create your own illustration that demonstrates the key themes of the article.

Oral

⇨ Why do complementary and alternative medicine practitioners often advertise their treatments as being holistic? Discuss as a group.

⇨ Make a list of so-called 'old wives' tales' surrounding ailments and remedies. Many of them are still talked about, if not believed, today. Are any of them grounded in truth? Discuss as a class.

⇨ As a class, debate the following statement: 'Homeopathy should be available on the NHS in all areas of the country.'

⇨ Create a PowerPoint presentation that explores the benefits and draw-backs of complementary medicine.

⇨ In pairs, discuss this extract from Tim Minchin's beat poem Storm (warning: full poem contains strong language): 'You know what they call alternative medicine that's been proved to work? Medicine.'

Reading/writing

⇨ Read *'I feel empowered, in control of my body': four women on fighting cancer with alternative therapies* (page 28-30) and *Complementary medicines may put cancer patients' lives at risk* (page 31). Write a short essay that discusses the pros and cons of cancer patients using complementary medicines.

⇨ Write a letter to your local MP explaining why you think homeopathic treatments should be available on the NHS.

⇨ Read *Pregnant women using alternative therapies urged to tell their doctors* (page 38) and write a summary of the article that could be reprinted in a GP's newsletter.

⇨ Choose an alternative treatment, such as acupuncture, and write a 'beginner's guide', explaining the history behind the treatment, what it is used for and how successful it is. Your guide should be no more than three sides of A4.

⇨ Choose one of the illustrations from this book, and write two paragraphs exploring what the artist was trying to portray with their image.

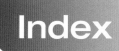
Index

acupuncture 2, 25
  and dementia treatment 21
  health and safety 9
  and palliative care 23
aloe vera 26–7
alternative therapies
  and cancer 6, 7, 19
  costs 19
  definition 18
  future of 5–6
antibiotic resistance 6
aromatherapy 3–4
  and dementia treatment 21
  and palliative care 23

back pain and acupuncture 2
Beddington, John 32, 34, 35
bright light therapy and dementia treatment 21

CAM see complementary and alternative medicine
CAMbrella Roadmap for European CAM Research 10
cancer
  and complementary and alternative therapies 6–9, 19, 28–30
  conventional treatment 7–8
  dangers of complementary medicines 31
Charles, Prince of Wales, and homeopathy debate 36
chelation therapy 4
chemotherapy nausea and acupuncture 2
Chinese herbal medicine
  and dementia 22
  and depression 24–5
chiropractic 3, 8
choosing a practitioner 8–9, 11, 21, 23
Choto-san and dementia treatment 22
Colquhoun, David 36
complementary and alternative medicine
  choosing a practitioner 8–9, 11, 21, 23
  definitions 6, 7, 18
  increasing popularity 5–6, 11
  regulation see regulation
  types 1–4, 6–7
complementary therapies
  and cancer 6–7, 19
  definition 18
  and palliative care 23
conventional cancer treatments 7–8
costs of complementary and alternative therapies 19
cranberries 27

Darwin, Charles 32
Davies, Sally 32, 34
dementia, complementary and alternative therapies 20–22
depression and Chinese herbal medicine 24–5

Eames, Sara 35
emotional benefit of complementary therapies 23

European Union
  and complementary and alternative medicine 10
  herbal medicines legislation 13–14, 15

faith healing 4
Flynn, Paul 36
foods and plants as natural remedies 26–7

garlic 27
ginger 27
Ginkgo biloba extract 22
Global Tiger Recovery Program (GTRP) 17
grapes 27

headaches, acupuncture treatment 2
health and safety in acupuncture 9
herbal medicines 4
  and dementia treatment 21–2
  and depression treatment 24–5
  regulation 13–14, 15
holistic treatment 11
homeopathy 1–2
  and the NHS 34–5, 36
  public opinions 32–3
  regulation 12
honey 27
Hunt, Jeremy 32, 34, 36
hypnosis 4

in vitro fertilisation and acupuncture 2
integrated healthcare 7
IVF and acupuncture 2

Kami-Umtan-To 22

legislation on herbal medicines 13–14, 15
light therapy and dementia treatment 21

macrobiotic diets 4
manipulative therapies see chiropractic; osteopathy
massage and dementia treatment 22
McCabe, Steve 36
MHRA (Medicines and Healthcare Products Regulatory Agency) and homeopathy 12
migraine, acupuncture treatment 2
music therapy and dementia treatment 22

natural remedies 26–7
nausea, acupuncture treatment 2
neck pain, acupuncture treatment 2
NHS and CAM 19
  homeopathy 34–5, 36
NICE guidelines on CAM 19

Acknowledgements

The publisher is grateful for permission to reproduce the material in this book. While every care has been taken to trace and acknowledge copyright, the publisher tenders its apology for any accidental infringement or where copyright has proved untraceable. The publisher would be pleased to come to a suitable arrangement in any such case with the rightful owner.

Additional acknowledgements

Editorial on behalf of Independence Educational Publishers by Cara Acred.

With thanks to the Independence team: Mary Chapman, Sandra Dennis, Christina Hughes, Jackie Staines and Jan Sunderland.

Cara Acred

Cambridge

September 2014

Images

Cover, iii, 22, 30 and 38: iStock; page 15 © John French; page 26 © Dominik Martin.

Illustrations

Don Hatcher: pages 8 & 12. Simon Kneebone: pages 18 & 34. Angelo Madrid: pages 5 & 32.